Acellular Dermal Matrices in Breast Surgery

Guest Editor

RICHARD A. BAXTER, MD

CLINICS IN PLASTIC SURGERY

www.plasticsurgery.theclinics.com

April 2012 • Volume 39 • Number 2

SAUNDERS an imprint of ELSEVIER, Inc.

W.B. SAUNDERS COMPANY
A Division of Elsevier Inc.

1600 John F. Kennedy Boulevard • Suite 1800 • Philadelphia, Pennsylvania 19103-2899

http://www.theclinics.com

CLINICS IN PLASTIC SURGERY Volume 39, Number 2
April 2012 ISSN 0094-1298, ISBN-13: 978-1-4557-3920-2

Editor: Joanne Husovski

Clinics in Plastic Surgery (ISSN 0094-1298) is published quarterly by Elsevier Inc., 360 Park Avenue South, New York, NY 10010-1710. Months of issue are January, April, July, and October. Business and Editorial Offices: 1600 John F. Kennedy Blvd., Suite 1800, Philadelphia, PA 19103-2899. Periodicals postage paid at New York, NY and additional mailing offices. Subscription prices are $448.00 per year for US individuals, $666.00 per year for US institutions, $221.00 per year for US students and residents, $509.00 per year for Canadian individuals, $779.00 per year for Canadian institutions, $578.00 per year for international individuals, $779.00 per year for international institutions, and $279.00 per year for Canadian and foreign students/residents. To receive student/resident rate, orders must be accompanied by name of affiliated institution, date of term, and the *signature* of program/residency coordinator on institution letterhead. Orders will be billed at individual rate until proof of status is received. Foreign air speed delivery is included in all *Clinics* subscription prices. All prices are subject to change without notice. **POSTMASTER:** Send address changes to *Clinics in Plastic Surgery*, Elsevier Health Sciences Division, Subscription Customer Service, 3251 Riverport Lane, Maryland Heights, MO 63043. **Customer Service: 1-800-654-2452 (US and Canada). From outside of the United States and Canada, call 314-447-8871. Fax: 314-447-8029. E-mail: JournalsCustomerService-usa@elsevier.com (for print support); JournalsOnlineSupport-usa@ elsevier.com (for online support).**

Reprints. For copies of 100 or more of articles in this publication, please contact the Commercial Reprints Department, Elsevier Inc., 360 Park Avenue South, New York, New York 10010-1710. Tel.: (+1) 212-633-3812; Fax: (+1) 212-462-1935; E-mail: reprints@elsevier.com.

Clinics in Plastic Surgery is covered in *Current Contents, EMBASE/Excerpta Medica, Science Citation Index, MEDLINE/ PubMed (Index Medicus), ASCA,* and *ISI/BIOMED.*

Printed and bound by CPI Group (UK) Ltd, Croydon, CR0 4YY

Transferred to Digital Print 2012

Contributors

GUEST EDITOR

RICHARD A. BAXTER, MD, FACS
Private Practice, Seattle, Washington

AUTHORS

OLUBIMPE A. AYENI, MD, MPH, FRCSC
Clinical Fellow, Division of Plastic Surgery,
Beth Israel Deaconess Medical Center,
Harvard Medical School, Boston,
Massachusetts

RICHARD A. BAXTER, MD, FACS
Private Practice, Seattle, Washington

BRADLEY P. BENGTSON, MD, FACS
Founder, Bengtson Center for Aesthetics and
Plastic Surgery, Grand Rapids, Michigan

ANGELA CHENG, MD
Breast and Microsurgery Fellow, Department
of Plastic Surgery, University of Texas
Southwestern Medical Center, Dallas, Texas

JOSEPH J. DISA, MD, FACS
Plastic and Reconstructive Surgery, Memorial
Sloan-Kettering Cancer Center, New York,
New York

LAWRENCE B. DRAPER, MD
Institute for Reconstructive Plastic Surgery,
New York University School of Medicine,
New York, New York

AHMED M.S. IBRAHIM, MD
Research Fellow, Division of Plastic Surgery,
Beth Israel Deaconess Medical Center,
Harvard Medical School, Boston,
Massachusetts

DAVID KAUFMAN, MD, FACS
Private Practice Plastic Surgery, Kaufman and
Clark Plastic Surgery, Folsom, California

PETER A. LENNOX, MD, FRCSC
Clinical Associate Professor, Division of
Plastic and Reconstructive Surgery,
Department of Surgery, University of British
Columbia, Vancouver, British Columbia,
Canada

SAMUEL J. LIN, MD
Assistant Professor of Surgery, Division of
Plastic Surgery, Beth Israel Deaconess
Medical Center, Harvard Medical School,
Boston, Massachusetts

SHEINA A. MACADAM, MD, MHS, FRCSC
Clinical Assistant Professor, Division of
Plastic and Reconstructive Surgery,
Department of Surgery, University of British
Columbia, Vancouver, British Columbia,
Canada

HUNTER R. MOYER, MD
Chief Resident, Division of Plastic Surgery,
Emory University, Atlanta, Georgia

JAMES D. NAMNOUM, MD
Assistant Clinical Professor, Emory University;
Private Practice, Atlanta Plastic Surgery,
Atlanta, Georgia

MICHEL SAINT-CYR, MD, FRCS
Associate Professor, Department of Plastic
Surgery, University of Texas Southwestern
Medical Center, Dallas, Texas

C. ANDREW SALZBERG, MD
Associate Professor of Plastic Surgery, New
York Medical College, Valhalla, New York

SUMNER A. SLAVIN, MD
Associate Clinical Professor of Surgery,
Division of Plastic Surgery, Beth Israel
Deaconess Medical Center, Harvard Medical
School, Boston, Massachusetts

BRUCE M. TOPOL, MD, FACS
Chief, Division of Plastic Surgery,
The Elliot Hospital; Plastic Surgery Staff,
Catholic Medical Center, Manchester,
New Hampshire

Contents

The use of acellular dermal matrices (ADMs) has become a useful adjunct to implant-based breast reconstruction and revision of the augmented breast. In both instances, the goal is replacement or reinforcement of thinned or missing tissues for implant support and control of the implant pocket. This article reviews the factors that contribute to periprosthetic tissue thinning, and the advantages and limitations of the use of ADMs for revision breast surgery and breast reconstruction. Proof of concept for the use of ADMs in the periprosthetic space is detailed from early clinical experience and histologic analysis documenting vascular ingrowth and cellular repopulation.

This article focuses on the contribution of acellular dermal matrices (ADMs) to immediate breast reconstruction. The current literature on ADMs is reviewed and the potential advantages and disadvantages of their use are highlighted. Technical considerations on how to effectively use these materials is presented.

The expectations for improved results in postmastectomy reconstruction for women have increased in the past decade. The modified radical mastectomy has given way to breast conservation techniques using principles of skin preservation. Skin-sparing and nipple-sparing mastectomies have allowed plastic surgeons to perform breast reconstruction with the advantage of an intact skin envelope. Acellular dermal matrix is a biotechnological tissue prepared from either human or porcine skin. During processing, the cellular components that cause rejection and inflammation are removed, producing a structurally intact tissue matrix that serves as the biologic scaffold necessary for tissue ingrowth, angiogenesis, and tissue regeneration.

Capsular contracture is one of the most common complications following breast surgery with implants and is a common cause for reoperation. Many techniques have been described to treat or prevent recurrent capsular contracture with varying success. Acellular dermal matrix (ADM), in combination with periprosthetic capsulectomy, is a powerful tool to delay or prevent recurrent contracture. Excellent results have been obtained when this approach has been used in patients with capsular contracture, but at increased cost.

Revision breast augmentation to treat implant malposition is fraught with challenges. This article focuses on treatment of implant malposition by using acellular dermal matrices (ADMs) with the intent of creating more reliable and accurate results. The article discusses the use of ADMs in patients with breast implant complications such as bottoming out, lateral implant displacement, or synmastia. ADM is a foreign material, thereby adding potential complications to consider.

This article examines the effects of radiation on prosthetic breast reconstruction when human dermal allograft is used in the reconstruction. A brief review of radiation terminology and techniques as applied to the breast is given, followed by a review of the effects of radiation on wound healing in human tissue. The effects of radiation on prosthetic breast reconstruction before the advent of dermal allografting are reviewed. The addition of dermal allograft in reconstruction has led to a reduced number of complications. An algorithm for surgical treatment of irradiated prosthetic breast reconstructions is presented, with a discussion of the authors technique.

This article explores whether some new acellular dermal matrices (ADMs) can be applied to breast augmentation or reconstruction revision, and particularly whether they can withstand the centripetal pull and prevent recurrent stretch deformities following periareolar mastopexy. Acellular dermis use in breast reconstruction and aesthetic breast revision is a fortuitous development, because their original purpose was for burn reconstruction. Although level 1 evidence remains lacking, ADMs have become integral adjuncts in breast reconstruction, complex hernia, and aesthetic breast revision. New applications continue to be explored, although these are in early stages of development and their long-term value remains to be confirmed.

This is a brief review of the history of the role of acellular dermal matrices in breast reconstruction surgery, with a summary of several currently available products, including a table of comparisons. Key features, including biologic tissue source, surgical preparation, sterility, polarity, contraindications, shelf life, and cost, are examined. A paucity of data exists to directly compare AlloDerm®, DermaMatrix®, Strattice™, Permacol™, DermACELL, FlexHD®, SurgiMend®, and ALLOMAX™ for breast reconstruction; most studies relate to hernia repair. An ideal acellular dermal matrix product is still unavailable but the information provided in this review should facilitate a breast surgeons decision-making process.

Acellular Dermal Matrices in Breast Surgery: Tips and Pearls

Olubimpe A. Ayeni, Ahmed M.S. Ibrahim, Samuel J. Lin, and Sumner A. Slavin

Acellular dermal matrices (ADMs) have been used for postmastectomy breast reconstruction, primary and secondary breast augmentation, and reduction mammaplasty. In postmastectomy breast reconstruction, ADMs can be used to either create an implant pocket in single-stage reconstruction or to create the inferolateral portion of the tissue expander pocket in two-stage reconstruction. Specific deformities after cosmetic breast augmentation such as contour irregularities and implant malposition can be addressed with ADMs. The use of ADMs is a safe alternative for the correction of breast deformities after reconstructive and aesthetic breast surgery.

Sheina A. Macadam and Peter A. Lennox

This article is a review of cost considerations and outcomes pertaining to the use of acellular dermal matrices (ADMs) in reconstructive and aesthetic breast surgery. The history of the use of ADMs in breast surgery and all case series describing outcomes and use of ADM in breast reconstructive and aesthetic surgery are reviewed. Weighted averages for clinically relevant outcomes for reconstructive and aesthetic breast surgery are provided. Cost considerations of ADM use in breast surgery are described and as an example, a single institution's experience with implementation of ADM into a preexisting breast surgery program, is used.

Clinics in Plastic Surgery

THE CLINICS ARE AVAILABLE ONLINE!

Access your subscription at:
www.theclinics.com

Current State of the Art for Acellular Dermal Matrices in Breast Surgery

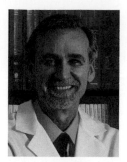

Richard A. Baxter, MD
Guest Editor

The use of acellular dermal matrices (ADMs) in breast surgery has been transformative over the past decade. For implant-related problems, they can provide a unifying solution to the multiple issues stemming from inadequate tissue for coverage and support. The concept of a living internal bra is a compelling one for patients and plastic surgeons alike. Challenging problems such as implant rippling, malposition, and capsular contracture have all found a potential solution with ADMs. Extending this concept to reconstruction, ADMs have helped define a new model. Along with increasing use of skin- and nipple-sparing mastectomy, the availability of BRCA genetic testing, and better implants, many patients now achieve superior outcomes with mastectomy than with "breast-conserving" treatment with radiation and lumpectomy. Many thoughtful innovators have contributed to these developments, and this issue of the *Clinics in Plastic Surgery* is dedicated to those forward-thinking surgeons.

Controversies remain and so I have encouraged the contributors to this issue to take a balanced view. Indications for use are not rigorously defined for every potential application despite the utility demonstrated by broad clinical experience, and prospective trial data where they exist often lack clearly delineated inclusion/exclusion criteria. This issue addresses the current state of the art with ADMs in breast surgery and I hope will provide some guidance as the science evolves.

Richard A. Baxter, MD
Plastic Surgery Clinic
6100 219th Street SW, Suite 290
Mountlake Terrace, WA 98043, USA

E-mail address:
drbaxter@drbaxter.com

Clin Plastic Surg 39 (2012) ix
doi:10.1016/j.cps.2012.02.008
0094-1298/12/$ – see front matter

Erratum

Skin Tissue Engineering—In Vivo and In Vitro Applications CPS Volume 39, Issue 1, Pages 1-102 (January 2012)

Florian Groeber [a,b,1], Monika Holeitera [c,1], Martina Hampel [a,b], Svenja Hinderer [a,c], Katja Schenke-Layland [a,c,*]

[a] Department of Cell and Tissue Engineering, Fraunhofer-Institute for Interfacial Engineering and Biotechnology (IGB), Nobelstrasse 12, 70569 Stuttgart, Germany

[b] Institute for Interfacial Engineering, Nobelstrasse 12, 70569 Stuttgart, Germany

[c] Faculty of Medicine, Eberhard Karls University Tübingen, Silcherstrasse 7, 72076 Tübingen, Germany

[1] Both authors contributed equally to this manuscript.

* Corresponding author. Department of Cell and Tissue Engineering, Fraunhofer IGB, Nobelstrasse 12, 70569 Stuttgart, Germany.

This article is a re-publication of an article previously published in Advanced Drug Delivery Reviews, Volume 63, Issues 4–5, Pages 193-404 (30 April 2011); doi:10.1016/j.addr.2011.01.005.

This re-publication was initiated by the Publisher and credited to the original journal.

The article has been withdrawn due to the accidental and unintentional assignation of a new DOI.

The Publisher regrets the inconvenience caused.

Acellular Dermal Matrices in Breast Implant Surgery: Defining the Problem and Proof of Concept

Richard A. Baxter, MD*

KEYWORDS

- Acellular dermal matrix • Revision breast augmentation
- Breast reconstruction • Implant capsule

Key Points

1. Acellular dermal matrices (ADMs) have been used for more than 10 years for revision breast surgery and primary reconstructive and aesthetic breast surgery.

2. ADMs may act as a template for tissue regeneration via vascular ingrowth, cellular repopulation, and tissue remodeling.

3. ADMs in revision breast surgery address problems stemming from periprosthetic tissue thinning such as implant malposition and visible rippling.

4. Implant-based postmastectomy reconstruction may be more stable and secure with the use of ADMs.

5. Breast implant–related problems often occur in combination.

6. More predictable and stable outcomes for revision breast implant surgery may be achieved with the use of ADMs in some circumstances.

OVERVIEW OF BREAST AUGMENTATION AND BREAST RECONSTRUCTION

Breasts are important in disproportion to their specific functional role in reproduction. Why this should be so, and why the human is the only species in which breasts are permanently enlarged is a question for anthropologists and social scientists, but the evidence is clear. For example, patients who undergo mastectomy experience measurable benefits in quality of life and overall well-being after reconstruction. Among these benefits are improved feelings of sexuality[1] and body image,[2] particularly in, but not limited to, younger women. A line of evidence is developing suggesting that patients who undergo mastectomy plus reconstruction fare better than patients who are treated with lumpectomy plus radiation in both quality of life and physical measures (arm edema, shoulder range of motion).[3] This suggests that the characteristics of the breast, and not simply the presence of a breast mound, are important; a breast hardened by radiation treatment may not necessarily be a preferable option to a reconstructed breast, provided that the reconstruction can be done with minimal morbidity and aesthetically pleasing results. Trends in recent years toward early reconstruction with implants supported by

---

Disclosure: Dr Baxter is a consultant and speaker for Lifecell, Inc. and Allergan Breast Aesthetics.
Private Practice, Seattle, WA, USA
* 6100 219th Street SW, Suite 290, Mountlake Terrace, WA 98043.
E-mail address: drbaxter@drbaxter.com

Clin Plastic Surg 39 (2012) 103–112
doi:10.1016/j.cps.2011.12.001

ADMs indicate that a shift in approaches to breast cancer treatment is underway.

Patients who undergo breast augmentation similarly accrue tangible rewards in life.[4] For these reasons, and others less easily discernible, cosmetic and reconstructive breast surgery occupies a central role in plastic surgery. The drive to build better breasts has fueled significant innovation in the 50 years since silicone breast implants were introduced. The number of breast augmentations and postmastectomy reconstructions have dramatically increased, with augmentation becoming the most popular cosmetic surgery operation in the United States in recent years[5] and breast reconstruction moving up to the top 5 for reconstructive procedures. Concerns about complications focused initially on the implants and led to improved design such as the use of a barrier layer to minimize gel bleed, more cohesive silicone gels, and greater variety of profiles for better matching of implant dimensions to each patient's anatomy. These improvements led to a more favorable attitude about breast implant safety.

Surgical analysis and planning have simultaneously advanced in sophistication, including tissue analysis,[6] optimization of muscle coverage with the dual plane,[7] and modifications.[8] However, certain problems inherent to breast implant surgery are inevitably magnified with the increase in the numbers of women undergoing implant surgery and a larger pool of long-term implant recipients. Despite advances in implant technology and surgical techniques, as many as 1 in 4 patients who undergo augmentation will have a reoperation within 4 years.[9] In patients who undergo reconstruction, reoperation rates are even higher, a point emphasized by the US Food and Drug Administration in a 2011 status update.[10] Of particular note are rates of reoperation for revision surgery, estimated at more than 1 in 3.[9] Revision often begets further revisions, pointing to the challenges of reoperative breast implant surgery and highlighting the inadequacy of traditional approaches. Although some would argue that problems of capsular contracture, implant malposition, visible rippling, animation deformity, and other issues are largely avoidable with proper technique and implant selection, the need for solutions to these problems remains. Given that changes in tissue-implant relationships can occur over a period of years, the need for revision surgery is unlikely to be reducible beyond a minimum that is yet to be determined.

The use of ADMs has become a useful option for many of these problems. Originally conceived as a dermal substitute for burn reconstruction, ADMs did not find early acceptance for that application, but began to be used for implantation for soft tissue augmentation or replacement in other clinical settings.[11] Volume persistence in the range of 80% to 85% at 22 months was reported for facial augmentation,[12] and static slings for correction of facial paralysis were noted to be stable even after radiation treatment.[13] Success with lip augmentation,[14] septal perforation repair,[15] and periodontal surgery[16] suggested a range of other possible uses. The concept of stable tissue support and/or enhancement could be extrapolated to applications in breast implant surgery.

CLINICAL EXPERIENCE WITH ADMs

With increasing exploratory use of ADMs in revision breast surgery, the indications for their use expanded (See cases in **Boxes 1** through **4**). The examples begin with early experience and progress to more recent examples of various clinical problems. Although they represent different applications, the underlying issues highlight the common denominator of inadequate soft tissue support.

RESULTS: HISTOLOGY AND PROOF OF CONCEPT

Because of concerns about the fate of ADM grafts in the periprosthetic environment, early use was conservative, limited to multiple small pieces rather than large ones. As a result, some cases had a partial improvement rather than a definitive repair, with patients requesting additional grafts. This outcome provided the opportunity to examine the grafts at intervals after initial placement. In every such case, a similar appearance was noted, with a glossy surface, complete volume retention (gross visual estimation), and bleeding when incised (**Fig. 1**A).

Documentation of the histologic behavior of ADMs established a foundation for proof of concept for their use in the periprosthetic compartment.[17] Biopsies at 6 months revealed organized collagen with intact vascular channels, active fibroblasts, and a lack of scarring and inflammation (see **Fig. 1**B–D). The first available product, AlloDerm®, is derived from human donors and processed to minimize alteration of the extracellular matrix. The presence of an intact collagen scaffold along with matrix glycoproteins and cytokines are thought to be important factors in enabling cellular repopulation and long-term stability. The methods used to decellularize the matrix and/or sterilize it significantly alter the

Box 1
CASE 1: BREAST REVISION SURGERY AFTER BILATERAL MASTECTOMY

A 49-year-old woman presented after bilateral mastectomy for ductal carcinoma in situ and delayed reconstruction with an expander-implant sequence using saline implants. The expanders had been placed following satisfactory healing after mastectomies, using a dual-plane technique with muscle coverage superiorly and medially and pectoralis release inferiorly. The expansion phase was 6 weeks, reportedly without complications. A revision was done with capsulotomies and implant replacement several weeks after the expander-implant exchange. The patient's concerns were visible rippling, asymmetry, wide intermammary space, and unnatural contours. Because of an athletic lifestyle and personal preferences, the patient refused muscle flap procedures.

Directed examination showed a tall thin woman with a body mass index (BMI) of 20.5 kg/m². The implants were asymmetrically positioned with inframammary fold malposition on the right side and an intermammary distance of 6 cm. Tissue coverage was thin, with a pinch test of 5 mm on the upper pole (**CASE Fig. 1A**).

Given the patient's concerns, options were limited. A lack of tissue for implant support and coverage was determined to be the underlying problem, a condition that may be termed periprosthetic atrophy. In this case, the problem was amplified by implants of inadequate diameter (the options for implant profiles were limited at that time, which was before the introduction of high-profile or low-profile shapes.) Fat grafting was considered but there was a lack of donor volume and, although coverage may have been improved, this would not have added support. The use of acellular matrices in the periprosthetic setting had not yet been documented. However, based on limited but successful personal experience with augmentation revisions using ADMs, it seemed to be a reasonable choice among few options.

In conjunction with implant exchange and capsule revisions including bilateral medial capsulotomies and a right inferolateral capsulorrhaphy, a series of thick AlloDerm® grafts (Lifecell Corp., Branchburg, NJ, USA) was placed. The grafts were affixed with resorbable sutures, with 1 edge of the graft across the junction of the anterior and posterior capsule. The concept was to define the boundaries of the capsule, smooth the transition from chest wall into the breast mound, and improve coverage of the implant. Long-term results have been stable, with now more than 10 years of follow-up (see **CASE Fig. 1B**).

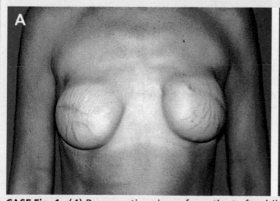 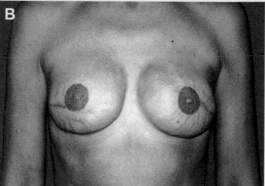

CASE Fig. 1. (*A*) Preoperative view of a patient after bilateral mastectomy and reconstruction with expanders and saline implants, and 1 revision. (*B*) One year after implant replacement and capsule revisions with acellular dermal grafts, and nipple reconstruction.

expression of growth factors as well as the ability of the matrix to support cell growth.[18]

ADMs seem to alter the nature of the capsule as well, a phenomenon that may be useful in dealing with capsular contracture (**Fig. 2**). A single cell layer membrane typically develops on the implant-facing surface over an ADM.

Cellular repopulation of ADMs has been extensively documented and further characterized.

Using a composite flap model based on the superficial inferior epigastric pedicle in the rat, Wong and colleagues[19] showed active host cell proliferation in the matrix as early as 7 days. In parallel with normal wound healing, endothelial migration continued for up to 14 days, by which time intact lymphatic channels were found as well. ADM sheets in the subcutaneous layer of the face are rapidly incorporated and maintain gross volume

Box 2

CASE 2: BREAST ASYMMETRY AFTER SALINE IMPLANT TRANSAXILLARY AUGMENTATION

A 26-year-old woman presented with significant asymmetry after transaxillary augmentation with saline implants (left 225 mL, right 410 mL). Her concerns further included symmastia (medial fold malposition) and bottoming out (lower fold malposition) (**CASE Fig. 2**A). Analysis of the problem determined a complex tissue deficit consisting of both a severe chest wall deformity, pectus excavatum, and a thin, lax soft tissue envelope for the breast, with a pinch test of 5 mm over the central mound despite submuscular placement.

Given the multiple problems in combination, traditional options were again determined to be inadequate. A supportive tissue envelope needed to be created to prevent relapse of the right implant across the midline, but muscle flap procedures were deemed inappropriate and capsule flaps insubstantial. ADMs had proved useful for more routine cases of medial fold malposition and so the concept was extended to this more challenging situation.

To have the option of adjusting fill volumes with patient input, the revision was done in stages using expander implants (Spectrum, Mentor Corp., Santa Barbara, CA, USA) and a solid silicone block behind the right implant. In addition, extensive capsule revisions were done including a superiorly based rectus abdominis fascia flap and two 4 × 7 AlloDerm® sheets placed medially and inferiorly as onlay grafts on the right side forming a sling to the pectoralis muscle. Fill ports were removed with a final volume of 375 mL on each side. Results are shown at 1 year (see **CASE Fig. 2**B).

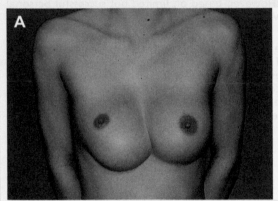 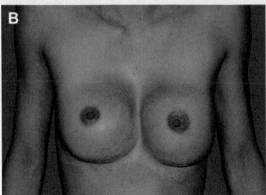

CASE Fig. 2. (A) This patient presented after transaxillary augmentation using saline implants; she now has asymmetry, and right medial and lower fold malposition, with underlying pectus excavatum and chest wall asymmetry. (B) One year after revisions including ADM grafts and adjustable expander implants.

over a period of months.[20] Expander-implant reconstruction using ADMs provides an opportunity for evaluation of the graft at the time of expander-to-implant exchange. A predictable take with less inflammatory response compared with native submuscular capsule was reported in a series of 20 patients having staged reconstruction.[21] Experience with this approach has now been well documented.[22,23]

Among the early concerns for ADMs in breast implant procedures was placement of a tissue-derived graft in a space with poor access to metabolic support, having a breast implant against one surface and capsule on the other. An autologous full-thickness skin graft in this environment would not be expected to be successful, given the metabolic demands of a cellular material. AlloDerm®

was originally developed for reconstruction of full-thickness burn wounds, in which circumstance the graft is placed with one surface on host tissue, with a dressing material on the outer surface. In the setting of the periprosthetic space, the hydrodynamics of the closed environment may even be theoretically advantageous. In an aseptic space with no risk of graft desiccation, circumstances may favor graft take.

It is now thought that acellular dermis occupies a middle ground, with no metabolic demands until cellular migration and vascular ingrowth occur. Immediately after implantation, it is neither living tissue nor prosthetic. In the absence of an inflammatory response, acellular dermis seems to be stable and metabolically inert, but, once integrated and transformed into living tissue, ongoing

Box 3

CASE 3: BREAST REVISION SURGERY AFTER SUBPECTORAL SALINE IMPLANTS

A 29-year-old fitness instructor presented for revision surgery after having subpectoral saline implants placed 7 years earlier. A year later, revision surgery had been done for malposition issues (details unknown). A deflation 3 years later prompted a replacement of both implants with 425-mL silicone gel high-profile implants. A capsulorrhaphy had been performed because of lower fold malposition with the first implants. The patient expressed concerns about severe rippling but was generally pleased with the size.

Directed examination showed a thin patient (BMI 21.7 kg/m^2) and significant traction ripples over both beasts (**CASE Fig. 3**A, B). Implant coverage over the upper pole was estimated at less than 1 cm by pinch test. Base diameter was measured at 13 cm.

Analysis suggested a problem of both coverage and support. With the implants already in the submuscular plane, additional options for coverage were needed, and with improved lower pole support the traction effect could be minimized. In a case of this severity, onlay grafts to the capsule in the upper pole alone are not certain to provide a definitive correction, and support to the lower pole alone may similarly be inadequate.

The surgical plan included replacement with moderate-profile implants (Allergan Style 15, 421 mL) and ADM grafting to all 4 quadrants (AlloDerm® thick, 4 × 7 cm). This created an implant pocket separate from the skin envelope. Six-month follow-up confirmed stable correction (see **CASE Fig. 3**C, D). The larger pieces of porcine-derived ADM available now would likely be a better choice.

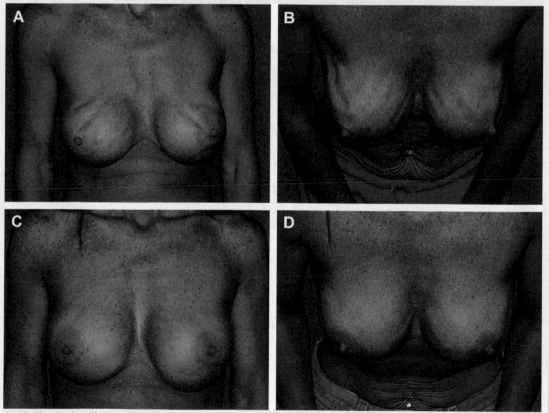

CASE Fig. 3. (A, B) Traction ripples in a patient with a history of saline implants, revision, then bilateral replacement with silicone gel–filled implants after a deflation. (C, D) Six months after 4-quadrant placement of ADM grafts.

Box 4

A 34-year-old gravida 3 woman presented 5 years after having subpectoral saline implants placed. Fill volume information was unknown but implants were reported to be 375 mL. The patient complained of rippling, a wide intermammary distance, animation deformity, lower fold malposition, and lateral malposition. She further requested an increase in implant size.

Examination confirmed these findings in a thin patient (BMI 20 kg/m²), with an intermammary distance of 4 cm and base diameter of 13 cm (**CASE Fig. 4**A). With flexion of the pectoral muscles, significant displacement of the implants with distortion of the breast shape was observed (see **CASE Fig. 4**B). Tissue coverage was estimated at 5 mm over the lower pole and lateral aspect.

At surgery, the pectoral muscle edge was mobilized from the anterior capsule (see **CASE Fig. 4**C). Cautious medial capsulotomies were done, along with an inferolateral capsulorrhaphy to create a pocket to accommodate a 450-mL high-profile implant with a base diameter of 12.4 cm. An elliptical ADM graft (Strattice™ Contour 2, Lifecell Corporation, Branchburg, NJ, USA) was used with 1 side affixed to the pectoral muscle edge and to the pocket along the inframammary and lateral folds to support the capsulorrhaphy. This concept of pectoral extension addresses the animation deformity by directing the force of muscle contraction away from the scar capsule while also improving implant coverage. Results were stable at 9 months (see **CASE Fig. 4**D, E).

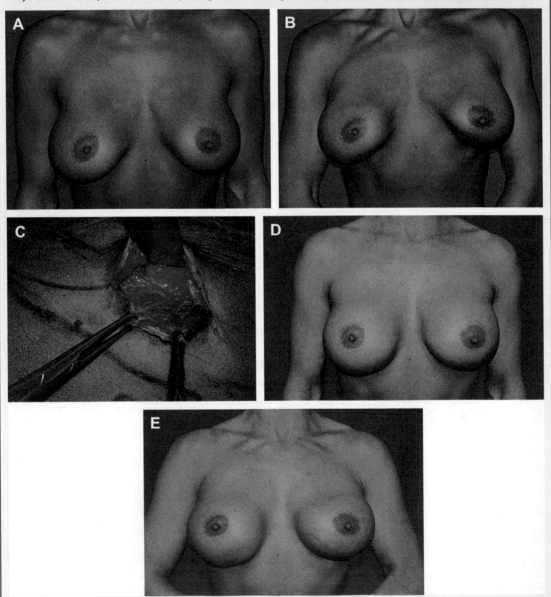

CASE Fig. 4. (*A*) Subpectoral saline implants with malposition, wide intermammary distance, and implant visibility. (*B*) Animation deformity shown with active muscle contraction. (*C*) Intraoperative view showing the anterior capsule dissected down to mobilize the pectoral muscle. The ADM will be sutured to the muscle along 1 edge, and the other to the inframammary fold. (*D*) Nine months after revision with Strattice™ Contour 2 graft (Lifecell Corp., Branchburg, NJ, USA) using the reconstructive model of pectoral extension. (*E*) Postoperative muscle flexion view showing amelioration of animation deformity.

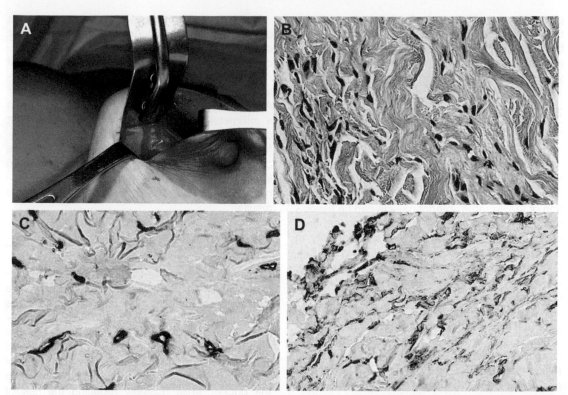

Fig. 1. (*A*) Gross appearance of a previously placed graft (appears as a white patch). (*B*) Hematoxylin-eosin stain of an onlay graft of ADM at 6 months, showing organized collagen and lack of inflammation. (*C*) CD34 stain for vascular endothelium documents vascular channels. (*D*) Vimentin stain shows active fibroblasts populating the graft.

remodeling can take place as with native host tissues. In optimal conditions, there is minimal, if any, apparent loss of graft volume over time.

The degree to which an unaltered matrix is important for graft performance remains a topic of deliberation. If altered through collagen cross-linking or sterilization processes that damage collagen or

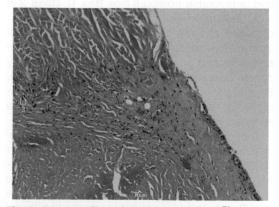

Fig. 2. Hematoxylin-eosin stain of a Strattice™ porcine-derived ADM graft at the transition to native capsule. Note the single cell layer over the graft (*left side*).

matrix glycoproteins, grafts may provoke an inflammatory response leading to encapsulation or resorption. Many such products are available now, although data comparing them with clinical results are scant.

DISCUSSION OF ADMs IN BREAST SURGERY

Few issues in plastic surgery have stimulated as much debate as the use of ADMs in breast implant surgery. Many of these issues are common to both aesthetic and reconstructive procedures. In both cases, reoperation rates for patients with breast implants have been of concern to surgeons, patients, and regulators alike. The need for early reoperative surgery is driven by several factors, a large one being simply a choice for a change in implant size rather than a complication per se, but a pattern becomes evident when considering the various contributors to implant problems leading to revision surgery: inadequate coverage and support. When these issues arise in the immediate postoperative period, they can be attributed in part to poor surgical planning or execution; in the long-term, there can be thinning of the tissues in response to the implant regardless of surgical planning and execution. This thinning of the tissues may be termed periprosthetic atrophy, but, in any case, the cause of the patient presenting with these conditions requires thoughtful analysis to obtain a lasting correction.

Tissue Deficit

The condition of periprosthetic atrophy represents a localized tissue deficit. In reconstructive cases with implants, the approach historically has been to attempt total muscle coverage, but this approach has been beset with difficulties. Elevation of the serratus anterior muscle can be associated with pain during the expansion phase, tight banding across the lower pole, and difficulty in controlling expansion vectors resulting in flattening and unnatural breast shape. Similar issues ensue from rectus abdominis elevation for lower pole support and coverage. The latissimus flap is a versatile workhorse option but is limited by potential donor site morbidity and scarring.

Inadequacy of the soft tissue envelope may be caused by several factors, either preexisting (the thin patient), surgical (mastectomy or reoperation), or a condition that develops gradually in response to implant-tissue interactions. In the thin patient, early results may be favorable but the tissues fail to provide support and coverage over time, and this may then progress to stretch deformity, traction rippling, or implant malposition. Options for definitive correction of these problems are limited because of the tissue deficit. With the concept of an internal bra, the use of ADMs addresses the problem by replacing a supportive framework.

Implant Dimensions

In some cases, implant dimensions exceed the compliance of the tissue envelope, the response being tissue thinning. For this reason, base diameter is a critical aspect of implant selection.[24] When implant diameter exceeds breast width, the anatomic boundaries must either be surgically violated, thereby hastening thinning, akin to the phenomenon of stress creep that is seen in other procedures in which tissues are placed on tension. Even without undue tissue stress, if the implant is too wide it must be radially constricted causing folding, which is manifest as ripples. Both factors contribute to long-term problems, but the former condition places direct pressure on the tissues as happens (albeit in a more controlled fashion) with tissue expansion. Once this has occurred, dimensional pocket reduction with capsulorrhaphy may be unsuccessful and does not address the issue of coverage.

Visible ripples may be seen even with an implant of appropriate dimensions. This rippling is most common laterally and inferiorly where there is typically no muscle coverage. The use of thin sheets of ADM for concealment of rippling in breast augmentation cases has been reported by Duncan.[25] Although these pieces are generally no more than a millimeter in thickness, control of the pocket dimensions and added support may be more helpful than coverage per se, particularly in the instance of traction ripples. Highly cohesive (form-stable) implants may be less prone to rippling but still require adequate coverage and support for optimal results.

Capsular Contracture

Another contributing factor is capsular contracture, the most frequent cause of implant reoperation surgery. If the severity of the contracture indicates a surgical approach, a capsulectomy is generally performed along with implant replacement and site change, which may further contribute to tissue thinning with potential loss of implant support. In this instance, the use of ADMs may serve a dual purpose of reinforcing the pocket while possibly reducing the risk of a recurrence.[26]

Combination Implant Problems

A common theme is how implant problems often present in combination. With periprosthetic atrophy, there is rippling, loss of support leading to fold malposition, either lower (bottoming out), medial (symmastia), or lateral, in various combinations. Because the underlying problem of periprosthetic atrophy manifests in disparate ways, patients often present with multiple problems in combination. **Case 1** represents what has become a classic example, with fold malposition, rippling, and unfavorable contours (see **Box 1**). **Case 2** is a more extreme example but, again, the condition of tissue atrophy on a foundation of chest wall asymmetry translates into complex combination problems and an artificial appearance caused by poorly disguised implant contours (see **Box 2**). By addressing the common issues with the use of ADM matrices, complex problems can be reduced to a more manageable concept.

The fourth case presentation represents not only the combination of problems (malposition, implant visibility, animation deformity) but the contributions of many who have advanced the techniques and the improved ADM products available now (see **Box 4**). In particular, the reconstructive model in which an internal bra is fashioned with fixation along 1 edge to the inframammary fold and the other to the released pectoralis muscle, has been useful in both implant-based reconstruction[27] and revision surgery for augmentation-related problems. Using the larger pieces now available, a total muscle-ADM pocket is formed that creates a unified approach to the multiple problems that tend to present together.

Another observation is the contribution of previous revision surgery, as in the first 3 cases. Each surgical intervention induces a new cycle of scarring and tissue stress, and subsequent attempts become progressively more challenging. This observation is illustrated by the statistics on revision surgery, the biggest predictor of which is a prior revision. An understanding of the tissue response to implants over time, and the effects of secondary surgery, leads to an appreciation of the underlying problem of periprosthetic atrophy.

Reflecting on more than a decade of using ADMs in breast surgery, a few themes become evident:

- One is the importance of breast reconstruction and breast aesthetics in general. Despite a controversial history, demand for implant surgery has continued to escalate. Perhaps for lack of good solutions, certain problems with breast implants were largely ignored, even while implant design and surgical techniques improved.
- Another theme that emerges is a reassessment of approaches to postmastectomy reconstruction, and even our approach to breast cancer treatment. The great push of the late twentieth century toward lumpectomy and radiation as breast-conserving therapy may now be giving way to skin-sparing mastectomy and immediate direct-to-implant reconstruction aided by an ADM internal bra. Comparative resource allocation, psychosocial impact, and patient morbidity are all being reevaluated in the light of developments in the past 10 years.

Looking forward, a motif of unifying significance appears. The use of ADMs represents 1 facet of the emerging field of regenerative medicine, the ability to fulfill the basic goals in reconstructive surgery of replacing like with like using scaffolds that direct tissue growth in specific ways. For example, ADMs have been explored as a template for seeding with adipose-derived adult stem cells, with demonstration of early penetration, proliferation, and expression of differentiation markers.[28] Tissue engineering acquires a new dimension with ADMs, beyond the two-dimensional concept of skin replacement or implant support. This concept is shown experimentally with a wound-healing model comparing healing with fibroblast-seeded ADMs versus ADM alone in rats. The filling of the defect as measured by magnetic resonance tomography was greater on the fibroblast-seeded side and the wounds had significantly increased breaking strength.[29] The effect persisted even in the presence of preoperative or postoperative radiation.

Nevertheless, the breast implant periprosthetic space represents a particular challenge, in that a tough but supple tissue layer is needed for implant support and coverage, but provoking too strong a tissue reaction may result in capsular contracture. The successful record of ADMs in this application, even though possibly lowering the incidence of capsular contracture, offers hope for the possibilities of regenerative medicine across a range of clinical needs. Lessons learned from early experience and proof-of-concept studies will help guide future work.

REFERENCES

1. Manganiello A, Hoga LA, Reberte LM, et al. Sexuality and quality of life of breast cancer patients post mastectomy. Eur J Oncol Nurs 2011;15(2): 167–72.
2. Medina-Franco H, Garcia-Alvarez MN, Rojas-Garcia P, et al. Body image perception and quality of life in patients who underwent breast surgery. Am Surg 2010;76(9):1000–5.
3. Freita-Silvas R, Conde DM, de Freitas-Júnior R, et al. Comparison of quality of life, satisfaction with surgery and shoulder-arm morbidity in breast cancer survivors submitted to breast conserving therapy or mastectomy followed by immediate breast reconstruction. Clinics (Sao Paulo) 2010;65(8):781–7.
4. Murphy DK, Beckstrand M, Sarwer DB. A prospective, multi-center study of psychosocial outcomes after augmentation with Natrelle silicone-filled breast implants. Ann Plast Surg 2009;62(2):118–21.
5. National clearinghouse of plastic surgery statistics. 2010 plastic surgery statistics. Arlington Heights (IL): American Society of Plastic Surgeons; 2011.
6. Adams WP. The high-five process: tissue-based planning for breast augmentation. Plast Surg Nurs 2007;27(4):197–201.
7. Tebbetts JB. Dual-plane breast augmentation: optimizing implant-soft-tissue relationships in a wide range of breast types. Plast Reconstr Surg 2006; 118(Suppl 7):81S–91S [discussion: 99S–102S].
8. Baxter RA. Subfascial breast augmentation: theme and variations. Aesthet Surg J 2005;25(5):447–53.
9. Important information for women about breast augmentation with INAMED® silicone-filled breast implants. Available at: http://www.accessdata.fda.

gov/cdrh_docs/pdf2/P020056d.pdf. Accessed June 11, 2009.

10. Update on the safety of silicone gel-filled breast implants (2011) – executive summary. Available at: http://www.fda.gov/MedicalDevices/ProductsandMedical Procedures/ImplantsandProsthetics/BreastImplants/ucm259866.htm. Accessed June 30, 2011.

11. Terino EO. Alloderm acellular dermal graft: applications in aesthetic soft-tissue augmentation. Clin Plast Surg 2001;28(1):83–99.

12. Constantino PD, Govindaraj S, Hitzik DH, et al. Acellular dermis for facial soft tissue augmentation: a preliminary report. Arch Facial Plast Surg 2001; 3(1):38–43.

13. Fisher E, Frodel JL. Facial suspension with acellular human dermal allograft. Arch Facial Plast Surg 1999;1(3):195–9.

14. Castor SA, To WC, Papay FA. Lip augmentation with Alloderm acellular allogenic dermal graft and fat autograft: a comparison with autologous fat injection alone. Aesthetic Plast Surg 1999;23(3):218–23.

15. Kridel RW, Foda H, Lunde KC. Septal perforation repair with acellular human dermal allograft. Arch Otolaryngol Head Neck Surg 1998;124(1):73–8.

16. Wei PC, Laurell L, Geivelis M, et al. Acellular dermal matrix allografts to achieve increased attached gingiva. Part 1: a clinical study. J Periodontol 2001; 71(8):1297–305.

17. Baxter RA. Intracapsular allogenic dermal grafts for breast implant-related problems. Plast Reconstr Surg 2003;112(6):1692–6.

18. Reing JE, Brown BN, Daly KA, et al. The effects of processing methods upon mechanical and biological properties of porcine dermal acellular matrix scaffolds. Biomaterials 2010;31(33):8626–33.

19. Wong AK, Schonmyer BH, Singh P, et al. Histologic analysis of angiogenesis and lymphangiogenesis in acellular human dermis. Plast Reconstr Surg 2008; 121:1144–52.

20. Scalani AP, Romo T, Jacono AA, et al. Evaluation of acellular dermal graft in sheet (Alloderm) and injectable (micronized Alloderm) forms for soft tissue augmentation. Clinical observations and clinical analysis. Arch Facial Plast Surg 2000;2(2):130–6.

21. Basu CB, Leong M, Hicks MJ. Acellular cadaveric dermis decreases the inflammatory response in capsule formation in reconstructive breast surgery. Plast Reconstr Surg 2010;126(6):1842–7.

22. Gamboa-Bobadilla GM. Implant breast reconstruction using acellular dermal matrix. Ann Plast Surg 2006;56(1):22–5.

23. Breuing KH, Warren SM. Immediate bilateral breast reconstruction with breast implants and inferolateral Alloderm slings. Ann Plast Surg 2005; 55(3):232–9.

24. Baxter RA. Indications and applications for high profile saline breast implants. Aesthet Surg J 2004; 24(1):24–7.

25. Duncan DI. Correction of implant rippling using allograft dermis. Aesthet Surg J 2001;21(1):81–4.

26. Maxwell GP, Gabriel A. Use of the acellular dermal matrix in revisionary aesthetic breast surgery. Aesthet Surg J 2009;29(6):485–93.

27. Spear SL, Parikh PM, Reisin E, et al. Acellular dermis-assisted breast reconstruction. Aesthetic Plast Surg 2008;32(3):418–25.

28. Ehsani N, Slack G, Fan K, et al. Adipose derived stem cells proliferate and differentiate on human acellular dermis. Plast Reconstr Surg 2011;127(5S):29.

29. Roessner ED, Their S, Hohenberger P, et al. Acellular dermal matrix seeded with autologous fibroblasts improves wound breaking strength in a rodent soft tissue damage model in neoadjuvant settings. J Biomater Appl 2011;25(5):413–27.

Do Acellularized Dermal Matrices Change the Rationale for Immediate Versus Delayed Breast Reconstruction?

Lawrence B. Draper, MD[a], Joseph J. Disa, MD[b],*

KEYWORDS

- Acellular dermal matrix • AlloDerm® • Strattice™
- Breast reconstruction • Tissue expander
- Implant-based reconstruction

Key Points

- Immediate breast reconstruction is a safe and reliable approach to breast reconstruction.
- Use of acellular dermal matrices (ADMs) does not necessarily increase the rate of tissue expansion or final fill volumes after immediate 2-stage breast reconstruction.
- ADMs are associated with an increased complication rate in breast reconstruction compared with traditional techniques.
- ADMs can be used in the setting of the irradiated breast.
- ADMs should be used judiciously in immediate breast reconstruction in the following situations: (1) eliminate dead space after nipple-sparing mastectomy; (2) insertion of the pectoralis major muscle is high, prohibiting complete coverage of the inferior and lateral aspects of the tissue expander with serratus fascia and muscle.
- ADMs may have an important role in direct-to-implant single-stage breast reconstruction.

OVERVIEW OF IMMEDIATE VERSUS DELAYED BREAST RECONSTRUCTION

Higher complication rates in immediate than in delayed breast reconstruction are reported in the literature.[1] Moreover, in many practice settings, coordinating immediate reconstruction with the breast surgery service and a busy operative schedule can be challenging. As a result, some practitioners are reluctant to incorporate immediate breast reconstruction into their practices. However, numerous reports have demonstrated safe and reliable techniques for immediate breast reconstruction with prosthetic devices. This article focuses on the contribution of ADMs to immediate breast reconstruction.

---

[a] Institute for Reconstructive Plastic Surgery, New York University School of Medicine, New York, NY, USA
[b] Plastic and Reconstructive Surgery, Memorial Sloan-Kettering Cancer Center, 1275 York Avenue, New York, NY 10065, USA
* Corresponding author.
E-mail address: disaj@mskcc.org

Clin Plastic Surg 39 (2012) 113–118
doi:10.1016/j.cps.2011.12.002

The current literature on ADMs is reviewed and the potential advantages and disadvantages of their use are highlighted. Technical considerations on how to effectively use these materials is presented.

Immediate Breast Reconstruction is Safe and Reliable

Since skin-sparing mastectomy was shown to be an oncologically sound procedure in the 1990s, implant-based breast reconstruction has become commonplace.[2] In 2010, 93,083 breast reconstruction procedures were performed. This number is an increase of 8% from 2009. Most patients underwent a 2-stage reconstruction with a tissue expander and implant (62,081). A significantly smaller number of single-stage, implant-only reconstructions (9452) were performed.[3] In the years ahead, the number of women who will undergo immediate reconstruction is likely to increase.

In a seminal article from 2002, Alderman and colleagues[1] published one of the first outcome studies on postmastectomy breast reconstruction. The article reviewed the complication rates associated with autologous as well as implant-based reconstruction over a 2-year period in 326 patients. The study concluded that immediate breast reconstruction, regardless of the reconstructive technique, was associated with higher complication rates than delayed reconstruction. With respect to implant reconstruction, the study examined 65 patients who underwent immediate reconstruction and 14 who underwent delayed reconstruction. The rate of major complications was 46% and 21% respectively ($P = .089$). Moreover, log regression analysis of major complications identified immediate reconstruction as an independent risk factor for developing a major complication with an odds ratio of 2.71. Many plastic surgeons continue to cite the report by Alderman and colleagues[1] as reason not to pursue immediate breast reconstruction.

In the intervening years, numerous studies have shown that immediate breast reconstruction is a safe procedure with a low complication rate.

Cordeiro and colleagues[4,5] reviewed a single surgeon's 12-year experience with early postoperative complications in 1522 reconstructions in 1221 patients. All patients underwent immediate postmastectomy reconstruction with a tissue expander, subsequent expansion, and a secondary procedure to exchange the tissue expander for a permanent implant.

Complications included:

- Hematoma
- Mastectomy flap necrosis
- Seroma
- Infection.

The observed overall complication rate was 5.8%. No increase in complications was noted in patients who underwent chemotherapy as part of their treatment regimen. However, the complication rate was higher in patients who had a history of chest wall irradiation. Review of the same cohort revealed that immediate 2-stage breast reconstruction yields good long-term aesthetic results with high patient satisfaction rates.[4,5]

What is Acellularized Dermal Matrix?

Many different products constitute the acellularized dermal matrix genre of implantable medical devices. The most commonly used and studied is AlloDerm® (LifeCell Corp., Branchberg, NJ, USA). AlloDerm® is cadaveric human dermis that has undergone a proprietary process to remove any antigenic properties of human skin. The end product is a biological matrix with the propensity to engraft into a vascularized tissue bed. It is not a sterile product, but it is aseptic, having been aggressively treated with a cocktail of antibiotic solutions to eliminate any organisms that may cause an infection. It comes in many different sizes and thicknesses, and has been described for numerous applications including:

- Abdominal wall reconstruction
- Static slings for facial reanimation
- Cleft palate repair
- Gynecologic and urologic reconstruction
- Breast reconstruction.

Other products include Strattice™ (LifeCell Corporation, Branchburg, NJ, USA), an acellularized porcine dermis. Strattice™ tends to be less elastic and resistant to deformational forces. One purported benefit of Strattice™ compared with Permachol (Covidien, Mansfield, MA, USA) is that Strattice™ is not cross-linked, theoretically allowing for more rapid neovascularization of the construct.

ADMs Emerge as a Popular Adjunct to Submuscular Immediate Implant Reconstruction

The first report of ADMs and breast surgery was for the treatment of contour abnormalities in cosmetic breast implant cases. Baxter[6] in 2003 described a series of techniques using AlloDerm® to correct difficult cosmetic problems such as synmastia, rippling, and malposition of implants. It was not until 2005, when Breuing and Warren[7] reported the use of AlloDerm® as an inferolateral sling in immediate breast reconstruction, that ADMs were identified as a useful tool in breast reconstruction. Breuing and Warren[7] described a series of 10 patients in whom AlloDerm® was used to augment a subpectoral pocket. The use of AlloDerm® allowed for a 1-stage reconstruction with tight control of the degree of lower pole fullness. The potential advantage of decreasing the amount of time needed for tissue expansion and the notion of improved contour of the reconstructed breast mound was also introduced. Salzberg[8] reported a similar technique used in 49 patients.

ADMs Have Many Perceived Benefits But Are Associated with Greater Complication Rates

Since these initial reports, the advantages of using ADMs have been highlighted in the literature and include decreased rates of capsular contracture and less postoperative pain; improved breast contour and camouflage of the implant; increased initial fill volume of tissue expanders in 2-stage reconstruction; 1-stage reconstruction with permanent implants.

Few of these claims are supported with prospective clinical studies. In addition, a randomized prospective study regarding the use of ADM and breast reconstruction does not exist. However, large retrospective cohort studies have provided some helpful observations. Preminger and colleagues[9] performed a matched-cohort retrospective study to investigate whether the use of AlloDerm® in immediate breast reconstruction affected the rate of tissue expansion or complications. Patients who underwent a 2-stage reconstruction with AlloDerm® did not have a greater rate of expansion than patients who underwent a 2-stage breast reconstruction without AlloDerm®. In addition, there was no significant difference in the rate of complications between the 2 groups. In this study, the investigators did not attempt to fill the expanders over aggressively in patients with or without ADM, which may explain the findings reported.

In a follow-up study, Antony and colleagues[10] reviewed the Memorial Sloan-Kettering Cancer Center experience with ADM in 153 2-stage breast reconstructions. The study revealed that advanced age, increased body mass index, and axillary dissection are independent risk factors for developing a complication in ADM/tissue expander breast reconstruction. Specifically, the ADM group had higher rates of seroma (7.2%) and reconstructive failure (5.9%) compared with the non-ADM cohort. Most cases of reconstructive failure were attributed to infection (3.3%).

These findings are confirmed by Chun and colleagues[11] in a review of 146 cases of ADM/implant-based reconstruction. Regression analysis showed that ADM use increased the risk of seroma formation more than 4 times and increased the risk of infection 5 times compared with a cohort who underwent non–ADM implant-based reconstruction. Although not statistically significant, Chun and colleagues[11] noted that mastectomy skin flap necrosis occurred with greater frequency in the ADM group. This finding was attributed to higher initial fill volumes and a tendency to retain more mastectomy flap skin in ADM/implant-based reconstruction. When cases of skin flap necrosis were excluded, a statistically significant increase in postoperative seroma rate was observed. However, the noted increase in the rate of major postoperative complications did not reach statistical significance. Thus, Chun and colleagues[11] concluded that seroma might predispose patients having ADM/implant-based breast reconstruction to infection.

ADM and Immediate Breast Reconstruction in the Irradiated Breast

In appropriately selected patients, neoadjuvant and adjuvant radiation therapy does not seem to preclude the use of ADM in immediate prosthetic breast reconstruction. Breuing and Colwell[12] describe their experience with 5 patients who underwent immediate tissue expander implant or implant reconstruction with AlloDerm®. All patients had adjuvant radiation therapy within 6 months of reconstruction and were followed for at least 2 years after radiation therapy was complete. None of the 5 patients developed capsular contracture or implant loss.

In a larger study, Spear and colleagues[13] reviewed their experience with 58 patients who underwent ADM augmentation of the subpectoral pocket in 2-stage breast reconstruction. Compared with dual-plane and more traditional submuscular techniques, the use of ADM was associated with a higher rate of seroma and infection. However, radiation therapy was the only variable shown to increase the risk of developing an infection. Based on these data, Spear and colleagues[13] concluded that a history of radiation therapy does not exclude patients from the use of ADM as part of their reconstructive regimen.

As stated previously, Antony and colleagues[10] showed that ADM use in immediate breast reconstruction can result in an increased risk of postoperative complications. However, multivariate analysis failed to reveal neoadjuvant radiation as an independent risk factor for postoperative complications. The investigators cited careful patient selection as a possible explanation for this observation. Specifically, they reported that candidates for breast reconstruction with tissue expanders and ADMs must have no evidence of radiation damage to the mastectomy skin flaps and were at least 1-year status post completion of radiation therapy.

Two-Stage Versus 1-Stage Breast Reconstruction

An advantage of using ADMs in breast reconstruction is the option of immediate breast reconstruction with permanent implants. As discussed earlier, AlloDerm® in this setting provides an extension of the subpectoral pocket and control over the aesthetic unit of the inferior pole.

One-stage breast reconstruction: Wise-pattern variation

Derderian and colleagues[14] describe a variation of Wise-pattern breast reconstruction that uses AlloDerm® and a vascularized dermal pedicle to improve breast mound shape and protect against implant exposure at the T-point of the mastectomy flap closure. In their study of 20 patients, a 25% T-point breakdown rate was reported. All the wounds healed with local wound care. Their study describes an innovative use of ADM and redundant local tissue to improve a previously described technique for immediate reconstruction. A caveat is that the Wise-pattern technique is only appropriate for patients with large breasts, who tend to have redundant skin after parenchymal resection. Generally, successful single-stage, direct-to-implant reconstruction with ADM requires well-perfused, viable mastectomy skin flaps, and a reconstruction that is similar to, or smaller than, the original volume of the breast.

Two-stage breast reconstruction

The example mentioned earlier shows the usefulness of ADMs in a single-stage technique. However, there are no prospective randomized clinical studies that compare the outcomes of 2-stage tissue expander/implant versus direct implant techniques.

The typical technique for immediate prosthetic breast reconstruction at Memorial Sloan-Kettering Cancer Center is a 2-staged approach. Immediately after mastectomy, a tissue expander is placed in a subpectoral pocket. After a series of expansions in the outpatient clinic, the patient undergoes exchange of the tissue expander for a permanent implant. Use of ADM occurs at the time of mastectomy and expander placement to elongate the pectoralis as an inferolateral sling. During the second stage, capsulotomy, capsulorrhaphy, and contralateral symmetry procedures are performed as needed.

Patients who have already undergone mastectomy and present for delayed reconstruction with tissue expanders and implants typically do not require ADM at the time of expander placement or exchange to the permanent implant. If the mastectomy flaps have previously been irradiated, delayed reconstruction almost always requires autologous tissue, with or without a prosthetic device.

Indications for ADM Placement

In the senior author's practice, ADM is used as an adjunct in immediate prosthetic breast reconstruction, not as a requirement. Most implant-based breast reconstructions can be performed using either total or partial muscular coverage of the expander, depending on the local anatomy and the quality of the mastectomy skin flaps. However, there is a role for ADM in prosthetic breast reconstruction to extend the length of the pectoralis major muscle when its insertion is high relative to the inframammary fold, particularly if the anterior rectus sheath has been violated during the mastectomy. In this situation, the distance between the inferior border of the pectoralis major muscle, anterior rectus sheath, and serratus fascia and muscle either prohibits complete muscular coverage of the expander or creates an excessively tight lower pole that is likely to result in a high-riding, taught expander that lacks adequate inferior pole projection. In this setting, ADM provides ample coverage of the lower pole, making up for the deficiencies in the patient's own tissues.

Nipple-sparing mastectomy has become a popular option for some patients. In this procedure, the skin envelope after parenchymal resection is frequently larger than a traditional skin-sparing mastectomy. As a result, it can be difficult to obtain full muscle coverage of a tissue expander inflated to a volume sufficient to preserve the shape of the skin envelope. ADM is used in this circumstance to allow for more fill in the expander and thus minimize dead space within the mastectomy skin envelope.

In single-stage, direct-to-implant reconstructions, ADM provides needed internal soft tissue support to allow an adequate-sized implant to be placed at the time of mastectomy.

Surgical Technique for ADM Placement

- Immediately after completion of the mastectomy, a subpectoral pocket is developed.
- A thick piece of adequate-sized ADM is hydrated in normal saline.
- The breast mound pocket is measured and the appropriate tissue expander is selected.
- The ADM is then sutured to the remnant of the inframammary fold inferiorly and the lateral aspect of the chest wall (lateral mammary fold).

- The ADM is trimmed as it is inset to tailor the inferolateral sling to appropriate dimensions.
- The tissue expander is inserted in the submuscular/sub-ADM pocket and the superior border of the ADM sling is approximated to the inferior border of the pectoralis major muscle with 2-0 vicryl suture.
- Before placing the tissue expander, the air is evacuated from the device and 60 mL of injectable saline are added.
- After placement, an additional amount of injectable saline is added depending on the quality and amount of mastectomy flap skin.
- One or two closed suction drains are left in the mastectomy space.
- Any obviously devitalized skin is resected before closure.
- Patients are given prophylactic perioperative antibiotics, typically until drains are removed.
- Drains are removed when output is <30 cc/24 hours (usually 7-14 days post operatively).
- Expansion begins ~14 days post operatively.
- Expansion continues every 1-4 weeks later-until complete.

Cost

A concern that many plastic surgeons have is the cost of incorporating ADM into breast reconstruction. Evidence suggests that the cost of a 1-stage reconstruction with ADM is similar to that of more traditional reconstructive techniques.

Janelle and colleagues[15] compared the expected cost of immediate implant reconstruction using ADM with a 2-stage breast reconstruction without ADM. The study took into consideration complication rate, capsular contracture rate, operating room time, and the cost of ADM. Their analysis projected that a 1-stage reconstruction with ADM is about $500 less than a 2-stage reconstruction with a tissue expander without ADM. The study has limitations. The analytical model was based on estimated cost at a Canadian university-based medical center. Cost estimates may be different in other health care systems. Moreover, in the model presented, if a direct-to-implant case takes 30 minutes longer than immediate insertion of tissue expanders, the cost advantage of the single-stage procedure is negated.

For a more detailed review of costs related to ADMs, see the article by Macadam and Lennox elsewhere in this issue.

SUMMARY

ADMs are a valuable addition to the armamentarium of the reconstructive surgeon. The advantages of immediate breast reconstruction are clear. Breast reconstruction should be tailored to fit the needs of the individual patient.

REFERENCES

1. Alderman A, Wilkins E, Kim H, et al. Complications in postmastectomy breast reconstruction: two-year results of the Michigan Breast Reconstruction Outcome Study. Plast Reconstr Surg 2002;109(7): 2265–74.
2. Toth BA, Forley BG, Calabria R, et al. Retrospective study of the skin-sparing mastectomy in breast reconstruction. Plast Reconstr Surg 1999;104(1): 77–84.
3. Report of the 2010 Plastic Surgery Statistics. ASPS; 2011. Available at: http://www.plasticsurgery.org/News-and-Resources/Statistics.html. Accessed August 1, 2010.
4. Cordeiro P, McCarthy C. A single surgeon's 12-year experience with tissue expander/implant breast reconstruction: part I. A prospective analysis of early complications. Plast Reconstr Surg 2006;118(4): 825–31.
5. Cordeiro P, McCarthy C. A single surgeon's 12-year experience with tissue expander/implant breast reconstruction: part II. An analysis of long-term complications, aesthetic outcomes, and patient satisfaction. Plast Reconstr Surg 2006;118(4): 832–9.
6. Baxter R. Intracapsular allogenic dermal grafts for breast implant-related problems. Plast Reconstr Surg 2003;112(6):1692–6.
7. Breuing K, Warren S. Immediate bilateral breast reconstruction with implants and inferolateral AlloDerm slings. Ann Plast Surg 2005;55(3):232–9.
8. Salzberg CA. Nonexpansive immediate breast reconstruction using human acellular tissue matrix graft (AlloDerm). Ann Plast Surg 2006;57(1):1–5.
9. Preminger B, McCarthy C, Hu Q, et al. The influence of AlloDerm on expander dynamics and complications in the setting of immediate tissue expander/implant reconstruction: a matched-cohort study. Ann Plast Surg 2008;60(5):510–3.
10. Antony A, McCarthy C, Cordeiro P, et al. Acellular human dermis implantation in 153 immediate two-stage tissue expander breast reconstructions: determining the incidence and significant predictors of complications. Plast Reconstr Surg 2010;125(6): 1606–14.
11. Chun Y, Verma K, Rosen H, et al. Implant-based breast reconstruction using acellular dermal matrix

and the risk of postoperative complications. Plast Reconstr Surg 2010;125(2):429–36.

12. Breuing K, Colwell A. Inferolateral AlloDerm hammock for implant coverage in breast reconstruction. Ann Plast Surg 2007;59(3):250–5.

13. Spear SL, Parikh PM, Reisin E, et al. Acellular dermis-assisted breast reconstruction. Aesthetic Plast Surg 2008;32(3):418–25.

14. Derderian C, Karp N, Choi M, et al. Wise-pattern breast reconstruction: modification using AlloDerm and a vascularized dermal-subcutaneous pedicle. Ann Plast Surg 2009;62(5):528–32.

15. Jansen L, Macadam S. The use of Alloderm in postmastectomy alloplastic breast reconstruction: part II. A cost analysis. Plast Reconstr Surg 2011;127(6):2245–54.

Direct-to-Implant Breast Reconstruction

C. Andrew Salzberg, MD*

KEYWORDS

- Breast • Implant • Surgery • Reconstruction
- Acellular dermal matrix

Key Points

- Direct-to-implant immediate reconstruction has created a paradigm shift in surgery
- Direct-to-implant surgery is easily reproducible in immediate reconstruction
- Direct-to-implant surgery has acceptably low complication rates
- The use of acellular dermal matrix (ADM) allows the surgeon to insert implants without undue stress on overlying skin
- Skin-sparing and nipple areola–sparing mastectomies are excellent indications for direct-to-implant surgery

---

OVERVIEW

The expectations for improved results in postmastectomy reconstruction for women in 2011 have increased in the past decade. The surgical treatment of breast cancer has evolved since the era of Halstead's radical mastectomy. The modified radical mastectomy has given way to breast conservation techniques using principles of skin preservation. The ultimate manifestation of this advancement can be seen in skin-sparing and nipple-sparing mastectomies. These innovations have provided plastic surgeons with the opportunity to perform breast reconstruction with the advantage of an intact skin envelope.

ADM is a biotechnological tissue prepared from either human or porcine skin. During processing, the cellular components that cause rejection and inflammation are removed, producing a structurally intact tissue matrix that serves as the biologic scaffold necessary for tissue ingrowth, angiogenesis, and, ultimately, tissue regeneration. ADM has been used extensively for soft tissue augmentation, including lip augmentation, depressed scar tissue repair, malar and submalar augmentation, rhinoplasty, and more recently for breast reconstruction.

In all these settings, the ADM has shown good incorporation, with excellent postoperative healing, no resorption, and minimal risk for infection, extrusion, hematoma, or seroma. In addition, because this tissue is acellular, it may have greater tolerance for ischemia because it has the capability to remain in place without breakdown until vascular ingrowth and cellular integration develops. This process can be shown by a biopsy of the ADM at 6 weeks after surgery (**Fig. 1**).

The Author's Use of ADMs

In 2001, I began to make use of the unique properties of ADMs to provide coverage for either an implant or a tissue expander in breast reconstruction, and I have relied on 2 important conditions as selection criteria when deciding which type of prosthetic device to use:

1. Vascularity of the overlying, postmastectomy skin envelope
2. Whether or not additional skin surface area is required to create a natural breast shape.

Significantly, skin-sparing mastectomy allows the reconstructive surgeon to focus on how best to

---

New York Medical College, Grasslands Road, Valhalla, NY 10591, USA
* 155 White Plains Road, Suite 109, Tarrytown, NY 10591.
E-mail address: asalzbergmd@yahoo.com

Clin Plastic Surg 39 (2012) 119–126
doi:10.1016/j.cps.2012.01.001

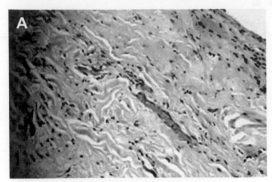

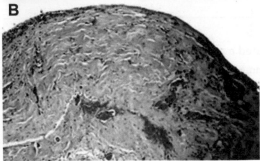

Fig. 1. Histology specimens of biopsied AlloDerm®. (*A*) Hematoxylin and eosin stain; (*B*) Verhoeff stain. These samples show replacement of the acellular tissue matrix with cellular ingrowth, revascularization, and capsular architecture.

replace the glandular volume without the restraint of providing donor skin of similar color and texture. The question of which reconstructive technique to use has also become more complex and the emphasis is now on choosing the appropriate procedure for each patient. The current surgical repertoire comprises prosthetic techniques using tissue expanders and implants, and numerous autologous tissue flaps, including pedicled flaps, free tissue transfers, and perforator flaps.

With the discovery of genetic markers of breast cancer risk, the demand and indications for prophylactic mastectomy have increased. Furthermore, patients are rightfully adamant that their choices include procedures with reduced operative time and postoperative recovery. To meet these challenges, potential techniques needed to provide a combined, single-stage approach for both the mastectomy and the reconstruction. For many patients, the benefit of using a prosthetic approach is the simplicity of the procedures as well as the avoidance of distant donor-site morbidity. The advantages of a single, direct-to-implant operation, particularly in the patient needing prophylactic mastectomy, became obvious, and such operations have developed into a viable alternative to the other, more

established reconstructive techniques. However, the surgical indications are specific and should be thoroughly familiar to both the surgeon and patient before selecting this direct to implant option.

Consultation for Direct-to-Implant Surgery

A comprehensive consultation with the patient before surgery is essential. This initial meeting provides the opportunity to review the risks and benefits of all reconstructive options as well as establishing candidacy for the direct-to-implant technique. This determination is directly related to the patient's body habitus, the ablative nature of the surgery, and the specific desires of the patient for contralateral breast symmetry. Patients who are able to have skin-sparing or nipple areola–sparing mastectomies are prime candidates. In addition, expectations must be reviewed and a realistic understanding of the pros and cons of the surgery established.

Indications for Direct-to-Implant Technique

Skin-sparing mastectomy is indicated in most patients with breast cancer who are also planning for immediate reconstruction. Prophylactic mastectomy may be offered to patients who present with a high risk with or without genetic markers for developing breast cancer or for the patient who is considering prophylactic mastectomy on the opposite breast. In either situation, a direct-to-implant technique can be used.

The ideal candidate for the direct-to-implant technique is a woman with a medium or smaller breast size, grade 1 to 2 ptosis, and good skin quality. Patients with a history of smoking are required to abstain for 4 weeks before and after surgery. Morbidly obese patients are generally poor candidates for implant reconstruction and are usually better served by an autologous option.

Contraindications to the Direct-to-Implant Technique

There are few contraindications to the direct-to-implant technique.

Considerations in patients undergoing radiation therapy

An important consideration is how to proceed in the setting of radiation therapy. If the patient has received prior postlumpectomy radiation treatment and the skin changes are severe with a firm and nonexpansive skin envelope, it is our practice to recommend autologous tissue reconstruction.

In our experience with those patients who have mild skin changes after receiving radiation therapy in the past, the chance of a vascular incorporation of the ADM in the radiated skin milieu is good, with an excellent indication for a successful outcome. A total of 40 patients in our series have received either preoperative or postoperative radiation treatments with no occurrence of capsular contracture, implant exposure, or infection requiring treatment.

In patients who are scheduled to receive adjuvant radiation therapy and who have declined an autologous tissue option, it is our practice to consider placement of a tissue expander in lieu of an implant. A pectoralis-ADM covering is created in the usual fashion. Expansion is performed rapidly with the goal volume reached before the initiation of the radiation treatment.

Skin viability

If there is any doubt as to the preoperative condition or intraoperative viability of the skin, then the procedure should be modified and an expander placed in the submuscular ADM pocket. A sufficient volume can then be injected into the expander; just enough to gently fill the skin envelope (hand-in-glove fit). In this way, skin tension can be avoided and filling of the expander can be performed once the skin has healed sufficiently.

In the past year, we have incorporated the use of intraoperative angiographic intravenous injection with the SPY (LifeCell Corp.) to assess the viability of the skin flaps after mastectomy and then after placement of the device. We have found that this technique not only provides instant feedback for the general/oncologic surgeon but also to the plastic surgeon who may see the effects of both the surgery and implant device on the overlying skin. The use of this technique in approximately 100 consecutive cases has predicted the final results.

Prophylactic mastectomy

A special consideration must be made for those patients presenting for prophylactic mastectomy who also desire a significant reduction in their breast size. In this situation, we do not recommend a nipple-sparing approach, because the viability of the nipple-areolar complex may be tenuous in the setting of a skin-reducing pattern or inverted-T incision. Skin pattern reduction, either vertical or Wise patterned, can be offered and used. Free nipple grafting has been performed in carefully selected settings with good outcome, but is subject to nipple loss from poor vascularity.

Preoperative Planning for Breast Implantation

As stated previously, the quality of the skin flaps after mastectomy is a critical component for a successful outcome. Choosing the appropriately sized implant to fill the space beneath these flaps is also an important consideration. See the algorithm in **Fig. 2**.

- We carefully measure the patient's chest wall dimensions and also use an array of sizers before surgery to gauge the anticipated volume that will be required after the mastectomy
- In addition, a three-dimensional volumetric computer program is routinely used
- In our experience, smooth, round silicone gel implants provide the best projection and shape
- A notable point is to choose an implant base width that complements the chest diameter, because a concave lateral chest contour results if the implant is not sufficiently wide.

We do not routinely recommend saline implants because they often produce an inadequate aesthetic shape and are prone to greater visibility and palpability.

There are many types of ADM available on the market today. See **Tables 1** and **2** for the allogenic and xenogenic biomaterials available now for breast reconstruction. The 2 major sources of skin use either a human or porcine model that is cleaved of cells and processed to create a framework of collagen into which cells can migrate.

The excellent experience with this graft in a wide range of soft tissue procedures has supported the rationale for its use in the postmastectomy setting where an inadequate muscular coverage exists. The potential for revascularization varies with both the source and thickness of the material. However, these materials have been used extensively throughout the body, significantly in abdominal wall and head and neck reconstruction.

DIRECT-TO-IMPLANT TECHNIQUE

It is our practice to interact closely with the oncologic breast surgeons and provide assistance in advance of and during the mastectomy. We strongly believe that there is a need for the plastic surgeon to be an active participant in the ablative surgery, thereby assuring the careful handling of the skin and the avoidance of traction injury to the flaps. This careful handling can minimize the stretching and distortion that can occur with retraction as well as lowering the risk of ischemic injury. If electrocautery is used for flap elevation,

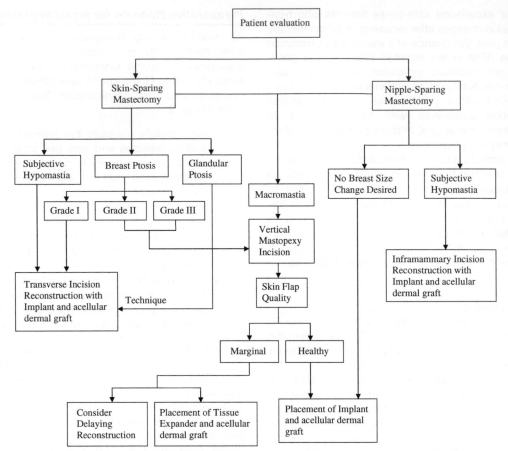

Fig. 2. Algorithm to guide clinical decision making in single-stage breast reconstruction with ADMs.

low settings are monitored to reduce the risk of tissue damage. The use of scalpel dissection or, more recently, radiofrequency devices (Peak Surgical, Palo Alto, CA, USA) for skin flap development is encouraged.

Using ADM to extend the submuscular plane, support the implant in its anatomic position, and define the inferior and lateral folds of the breast is critical for immediate reconstruction with the direct-to-implant technique. The operative concept was developed in 2001 and has proved to be successful in most cases.

- The technique begins by creating a subpectoral pocket extending from the second rib superiorly, medially to the origin of the pectoralis muscle at the sternum and laterally to the lateral mammary fold (**Fig. 3**).
- Elevation of a portion of the inferomedial muscle to allow anatomic placement of the implant is also performed.
- The ADM is sutured in a running fashion to the pectoralis muscle along its lower course from medial to lateral and then around and down to the lateral mammary fold (**Fig. 4**).

Table 1
Allogenic biologic materials currently available for breast reconstruction

Name	Company	Source Tissue
DermaMatrix®	MTF(Synthes)	Allograft
Flex HD®	MTF(Ethicon)	Allograft
NeoForm®	Tutogen(Mentor)	Allograft
AlloDerm®	LifeCell	Allograft

Table 2
Xenogenic biologic materials currently available for breast reconstruction

Name	Company	Source Tissue
Strattice™	LifeCell	Xenograft
SurgiMend®	TEI Biosciences	Xenograft
Veritas®	Synovis	Xenograft

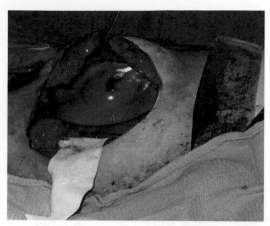

Fig. 3. Retropectoral pocket and raising of pectoralis muscle to allow insertion of implant and AlloDerm® placement to cover reconstructed breast and allow closure of skin flaps.

- No elevation of muscle is necessary at the serratus margins and direct suturing of the ADM with absorbable suture material defines and sets the fold.
- The appropriately sized implant (selected with the patient during consultation using three-dimensional imaging and trial sizes) is confirmed by surgical judgment as well as by the weight of the mastectomy specimen. If desired, a modest overcorrection is added to the final implant volume to accommodate the anticipated release of the skin elasticity following the mastectomy.
- After placing the implant between the muscle above, and the ADM below, suturing of the ADM directly to the inframammary fold

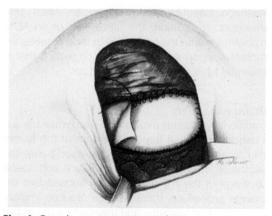

Fig. 4. Running sutures are used to secure the graft to the elevated lateral border of the pectoralis major on one side and to the serratus anterior muscle on the other side. (*From* Salzberg A. Non expansive immediate breast reconstruction using human acellular tissue matrix graft (AlloDerm). Ann Plast Surg 2006;57:1, Lippincott Williams & Wilkins; with permission.)

(IMF) at its desired position, without expecting migration, is performed (see **Fig. 4**).

- Two suction drains are placed, 1 in the subpectoral space and the other in the subcutaneous space.
- A hand-in-glove fit is expected with no dead space, and direct conformation to the lower pole decreases the chance of seroma formation.
- A perfect shape should be achieved at this point and postoperative settling should not be planned.

This technique has withstood the test of time, with patients' long-term results yielding little change in the last 10 years.

Figs. 5 and **6** show examples of patients before and after surgery.

Postoperative Care for Breast Implant Surgery

Typically, the patient remains in the hospital for approximately 48 hours. On discharge, the drains, which are covered with Bio-Patch (Johnson & Johnson, New Brunswick, NJ, USA) and occlusive dressings, are maintained for 7 to 14 days, with removal determined by the amount and quality of their output. A supportive surgical bra with an additional superior pole pectoralis strap is worn for 3 to 6 weeks to assist in the optimal positioning of the implants in the pocket. The patients are encouraged to perform moderate exercise to improve their arm range of motion, and to perform gentle massaging to prevent the development of axillary contracture.

Complications and Outcomes of Direct-to-Implant Surgery

Minor complications include:

- Suture exposure
- Wound healing delay
- Noninfectious skin erythema, which may occur in up to 10% of patients.

Major complications are infrequent, with:

- Seroma (1%)
- Skin necrosis requiring reoperation (2.4%)
- Hematoma (0.6%)
- Capsular contracture (0.2%).

Discussion on Breast Implant Technique

The selection of a breast reconstruction technique depends on individual patients' anatomy as well as their preferences. In general, the choice has been either autologous tissue transfer; usually the TRAM (transverse rectus abdominis myocutaneous) flap

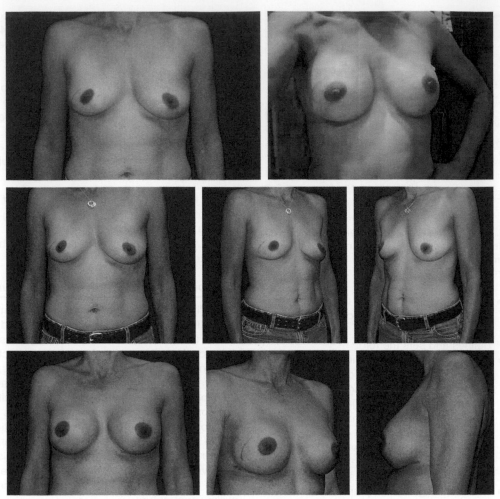

Fig. 5. (*Left*) preoperative and (*right*) postoperative views of the breasts following immediate direct-to-implant reconstruction with ADM.

or the expander-implant approach. Although these techniques represent significant advances in the management of the postmastectomy patient, they are not without limitations and complications. Autologous tissue reconstruction has the concern of donor-site morbidity; the expansion patient must commit to multiple visits to the physician's office for saline injections and, when the inflation is complete, a second surgical procedure is needed to replace the expander with a permanent implant (or, if a combination implant device is used, to remove the filling port).

Skin-sparing technique

In the past 10 years, skin-sparing techniques have allowed surgical oncologists to spare more skin, preserve muscle fascia, and perform nipple-sparing prophylactic surgery for high-risk or early stage patients. With the advent of the skin-sparing mastectomy, plastic surgeons have been given the opportunity to take advantage of the

aesthetic benefits bestowed by an intact skin envelope. In addition, the placement of an ADM in continuity with the pectoralis muscle establishes implant support and permits the projection that is essential for a natural breast contour.

Tissue expanders

Traditionally, a tissue expander is used when there is a need to increase the surface area of the breast skin. In addition, the expander is placed below the pectoralis muscle to assure sufficient soft tissue coverage of the implant. After the subsequent exchange procedure, this coverage reduces implant palpability and visibility, and maintains a protective barrier between the implant and skin. The routine use of tissue substitutes to cover expanders has now become a useful supplement and the attachment of incorporated ADM to the pectoralis muscle can provide a durable line of defense against thin skin flaps and potential exposure.

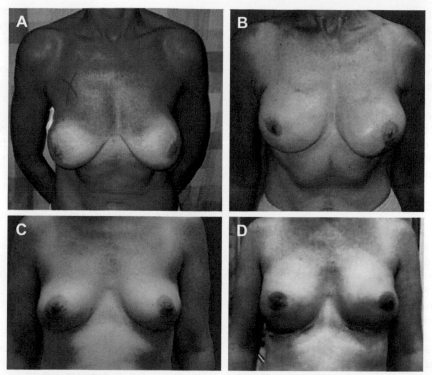

Fig. 6. Preoperative and postoperative views of the breasts of two women following immediate reconstruction supported by AlloDerm® grafting show good symmetry and desired breast projection. (*A*) Preoperative. (*B*) At 3 months after surgery. (*C*) Preoperative. (*D*) At 1 week after surgery.

Direct to implant with ADM

The technique of direct-to-implant reconstruction with ADM has expanded the surgeon's repertoire and given the patient an opportunity to have a 1-stage option (in a nipple-sparing mastectomy) that was previously available only when using autologous tissue. This alternative has become particularly attractive to young women with a genetic disposition to breast cancer. Those with insufficient available tissue for a flap can elect to undergo a nipple-sparing mastectomy combined with the direct-to-implant approach. We find that an inframammary approach to prophylactic mastectomy is reliable and gives the best cosmetic result. This technique affords patients the opportunity to receive a reconstruction with as little external scarring as possible (**Fig. 7**).

Personal experience with direct-to-implant reconstruction began in 2001 and now includes approximately 700 immediate direct-to-implant breast reconstructions in 460 patients. Before this, the expander-implant technique was, in most cases, the method of choice for immediate, prosthetic breast reconstruction. That approach allowed the available tissue coverage to be slowly increased for effective mound replacement. Incorporating ADM now provides additional coverage at

the serratus/pectoralis muscle interval and allows the immediate creation of the breast mound. The technique produces total implant coverage without the need for expansion, repetitive surgeries, and delayed return of normal body image. The success observed with the direct to implant with ADM technique indicates the effectiveness of the procedure as well as the long-term safety and aesthetic benefits of the approach.

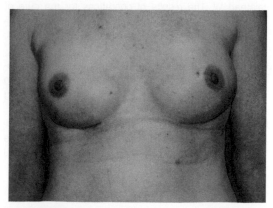

Fig. 7. Postoperative result showing incisions along the IMFs.

The direct to implant with ADM technique has created a paradigm shift allowing postmastectomy breasts to resemble the results achieved with aesthetic augmentation. With the ability to define the surgical implant pocket, support the device in the proper position, and reduce postoperative visits and the need for a secondary surgery, a new reality has been achieved. The use of a biologic product that is incorporated into the patient's own tissue ensures the benefits of regenerative medicine and eliminates encapsulation of nonbiologic material.

SUGGESTED READINGS

Alderman AK, Wilkins EG, Kim HM, et al. Complications in postmastectomy breast reconstruction: two year results of the Michigan breast reconstruction outcome study. Plast Reconstr Surg 2002;109:2265.

Ashikari RH, Ashikari AY, Kelemen PR, et al. Subcutaneous mastectomy and immediate reconstruction for prevention of breast cancer for high-risk patients. Breast Cancer 2008;15(3):185–91.

Birdsell DC, Jenkins H, Berkel H. Breast cancer diagnosis and survival in women with and without breast implants. Plast Reconstr Surg 1993;92(5):795–800.

Dean C, Chetty U, Forrest AP. Effects of immediate breast reconstruction on psychosocial morbidity after mastectomy. Lancet 1983;1:459–62.

Duncan DI. Correction of implant rippling using allograft dermis. Aesthet Surg J 2001;21(1):81–4.

Foster RD, Esserman LJ, Anthony JP, et al. Skin-sparing mastectomy and immediate breast reconstruction: a prospective cohort study for the treatment of advanced stages of breast carcinoma. Ann Surg Oncol 2002;9:462–6.

Gibney J. The long-term results of tissue expansion for breast reconstruction. Clin Plast Surg 1987;14:509–18.

Gryskiewicz JM, Rohrich RJ, Regan BJ. The use of Allo-Derm for the correction of nasal contour deformities. Plast Reconstr Surg 2001;107:561.

Halstead W. The results of operations for the cure of cancer of the breast performed at The Johns Hopkins Hospital from June 1889 to January 1894. Johns Hopkins Bull 1894;4:297.

Johnson CH, Van Heerden JA, Donohue JH, et al. Oncological aspects of immediate breast reconstruction following mastectomy for malignancy. Arch Surg 1989;124:819–24.

Jones FR, Schwartz BM, Silverstein P. Use of a nonimmunogenic acellular dermal allograft for soft tissue augmentation: a preliminary report. Aesthet Surg J 1996;16:196–201.

Kroll SS, Ames F, Singletary SE, et al. The oncologic risks of skin preservation at mastectomy when combined with immediate reconstruction of the breast. Surg Gynecol Obstet 1991;172:17–20.

Kroll SS, Coffey JA Jr, Winn RJ, et al. A comparison of factors affecting aesthetic outcomes of TRAM flap breast reconstructions. Plast Reconstr Surg 1995;96:860–4.

Kroll SS, Schusterman MA, Tadjalli HE, et al. Risk of recurrence after treatment of early breast cancer with skin-sparing mastectomy. Ann Surg Oncol 1997;4:193–7.

Losken A, Carlson GW, Bostwick J III, et al. Trends in unilateral breast reconstruction and management of the contralateral breast: the Emory experience. Plast Reconstr Surg 2002;110:89–97.

Menon NG, Rodriguez ED, Byrnes CK, et al. Revascularization of human acellular dermis in full-thickness abdominal wall reconstruction in the rabbit model. Ann Plast Surg 2003;50:523.

Miller MJ. Immediate breast reconstruction. Clin Plast Surg 1998;25:145–56.

Rohrich RJ, Regan BJ, Adams WP, et al. Early results of vermilion lip augmentation using acellular allogeneic dermis: an adjunct in facial rejuvenation. Plast Reconstr Surg 2000;105:409–17.

Salzberg CA. Nonexpansive immediate breast reconstruction using human acellular tissue matrix graft (AlloDerm). Ann Plast Surg 2006;57(1):707–11.

Spencer KW. Significance of the breast to the individual and society. Plast Surg Nurs 1996;16:131–2.

Stevens LA, McGrath MH, Druss RG, et al. The psychological impact of immediate breast reconstruction for women with early breast cancer. Plast Reconstr Surg 1984;73:619–28.

Stolier AJ, Wang J. Terminal duct lobular units are scarce in the nipple: implications for prophylactic nipple-sparing mastectomy. Ann Surg Oncol 2008;15(2):438–42.

Terino EO. AlloDerm acellular dermal graft: applications in aesthetic and reconstructive soft tissue augmentation. In: Klein AW, editor. Tissue augmentation in clinical practice. Marcel Dekker; 1998. p. 349–77.

Wainwright D, Madden M, Luterman A, et al. Clinical evaluation of an acellular allograft dermal matrix in full-thickness burns. J Burn Care Rehabil 1996;17:124–36.

Wainwright D. Use of an acellular allograft dermal matrix (AlloDerm) in the management of full-thickness burns. Burns 1995;21:243–8.

Wellisch DK, Schain WS, Noone RB, et al. Psychosocial correlates of immediate versus delayed breast reconstruction. Am J Psychol 1985;76:713–8.

The Role of Acellular Dermal Matrix in the Treatment of Capsular Contracture

James D. Namnoum, MD[a],*, Hunter R. Moyer, MD[b]

KEYWORDS

- Acellular dermal matrix • Capsular contracture
- Silicone breast implants • Silicone gel
- Breast augmentation • Breast reconstruction
- Capsulectomy

Key Points

1. Capsular contracture is the most frequent cause for device-related reoperation in patients undergoing breast augmentation and revision augmentation, and the second most common reason for reoperation following reconstruction.

2. Many established techniques have been described to reduce or prevent recurrent capsular contracture, but they are not effective in all cases.

3. Acellular dermal matrix (ADM) in combination with capsulectomy can prevent or delay recurrent capsular contracture.

4. The mechanism by which recurrent contracture is inhibited is not clear but may involve a delay of inflammatory cell infiltrate into the matrix (including myofibroblasts) modulating the foreign body reaction around the implant or a biomechanical interruption of the spherical contracture process.

5. More than 1 type of ADM has been shown to be effective at preventing recurrent capsular contracture.

6. More data are needed to determine whether the inhibition of capsular contracture in the setting of ADM and implants is permanent, and to identify the critical accompanying steps necessary to ensure lasting success from recurrent contracture.

Capsular contracture remains the most frequent device-related complication of breast surgery with implants and has been an intractable problem since the introduction of the silicone breast implant in the 1960s. The ongoing, prospective premarket approval trials of the 2 largest manufacturers of these devices Allergan (Irvine, CA, USA) and Mentor (Santa Barbara, CA, USA) with a follow-up rate of 67% to 92% have shown an incidence of capsular contracture ranging from

---

James D. Namnoum, MD is a shareholder and consultant, Allergan Corporation and Alure Medical.
Hunter R. Moyer has nothing to disclose.
[a] Private Practice, Atlanta Plastic Surgery, Emory University, 975 Johnson Ferry Road, Suite 100, Atlanta, GA 30319, USA
[b] Division of Plastic Surgery, Emory University, 975 Johnson Ferry Road, Suite 100, Atlanta, GA 30342, USA
* Corresponding author.
E-mail address: jdnamnoum@atlplastic.com

Clin Plastic Surg 39 (2012) 127–136
doi:10.1016/j.cps.2012.02.005
0094-1298/12/$ – see front matter © 2012 Elsevier Inc. All rights reserved.

9.8% to 14.8% for primary augmentation, 20.5% to 22.4% for revision augmentation, and 13.7 to 15.9% for primary reconstruction. Capsular contracture is the most common reason for reoperation in these patients (14.5% to 35.2%) and appears to increase with time.[1,2]

ETIOLOGY OF CAPSULAR CONTRACTURE

All implanted materials failing to acquire a blood supply incite a prototypical foreign body reaction characterized by the development of a scar interface between the foreign body and its biologic environment. Because breast implants are compliant as opposed to other implanted devices such as pacemakers or total joints, an exuberant foreign body reaction that becomes contractile around the implant will lead to deformity and pain. The resulting capsular contracture may prompt a need for reoperation, complicating the result and leading to additional recovery and expense.

Several factors have been associated with an increased risk for capsular contracture, including:

- Subclinical infection with biofilm[3]
- Silicone versus saline implants[4]
- Smooth versus textured surfaces[5,6]
- Subglandular versus subpectoral positioning[7]
- Postoperative hematoma[8]
- Silicone breast implant ruptures[9]
- Reoperative implant surgery[1,2]
- Radiation therapy proceeding or following reconstruction with implants.[10–14]

Pathogenesis of Capsular Contracture

Capsular contracture appears to appear at two different times:

1. Early, thought to result from poor sterility or surgical technique
2. Late, as a result of a chronic inflammatory process.

In either case, the exact biologic processes leading to the development of a thick, contracting capsule is unclear. Evidence from a variety of sources has implicated the activation of the fibroblast into a contractile myofibroblast as the critical event in the contracture process.

Myofibroblasts

Myofibroblasts have been noted in the capsules around breast implants since the 1970s.[15] Early in vitro studies of capsular tissue demonstrated a prototypical response to smooth muscle agonists and antagonists similar to that expected from smooth muscle preparations.[16] In Hinz's description,[17] fibroblasts differentiate into activated myofibroblasts with potent contractile properties conferred from α smooth muscle actin (SMA) in a 2- step process under the direction of transforming growth factor beta (TGFβ1), specialized extra cellular matrix (ECM) proteins like fibronectin, and the mechanical microenvironment.

Smad Signaling

Smad signaling is the major pathway through which TGFβ1 regulates expression of α-SMA in fibroblasts. In an experimental model comparing wild-type and knockout mice lacking Smad, irradiation caused thick, distorted capsules in the wild-type mouse but not the knockout mice, presumably due to inhibition of TGFβ.[18] Zinman and colleagues[19] demonstrated that rats treated with the angiotension-converting enzyme inhibitor enalapril, a potent inhibitor of TGFβ1, had significantly less peri-prosthetic fibrosis than untreated animals presumably due in part to the role TGFβ1 plays in activation of fibroblasts to myofibroblasts.

Stress Shielding

The mechanical microenvironment also plays a role in myofibroblast differentiation due to alteration in ECM stiffness. According to Hinz,[17] fibroblasts residing in intact tissues are stress shielded by normal ECM. With trauma or repetitive injury, increasing ECM stiffness provides a strong mechanical signal, inducing the formation of α–SMA negative stress fibers that persist until the normalization of matrix compliance. Factors that antagonize TGFβ1, normalize matrix compliance, and improve cell-to-cell contact down-regulate α–SMA in vitro; decreasing gel stress in vitro, a model for stress shielding, causes myofibroblast apoptosis.

Evidence that Acellular Dermal Matrix Plays a Useful Role in the Treatment of Capsular Contracture

Salzberg demonstrated an incidence of capsular contracture of 0.4% in review of his direct-to-implant immediate breast reconstruction in 466 breasts using ADM with 21 month follow-up including 0% contracture following irradiation.[20]

Maxwell showed a 0% incidence of capsular contracture at 1 year postoperatively following ADM use for revisionary breast surgery.[21]

Stump demonstrated the absence of capsule formation around implants covered in ADM in a primate model at 10 weeks with a significant decrease in myofibroblast staining in the ADM-covered implants as compared with the capsules in implants not covered with ADM.[22]

Basu demonstrated significantly decreased inflammatory response in biopsies of ADM as compared with native capsule around expanders at the time of second-stage exchange, suggesting that ADM potentially delayed the process of capsule formation.[23]

Technique for Correction of Capsular Contracture with ADM

There is no consensus as to the required steps to optimize the results for preventing or delaying the recurrence of capsular contracture when ADM is used. In a retrospective review, Collis[24] demonstrated a significantly lower incidence of recurrent subglandular contracture when total capsulectomy was performed rather than anterior capsulectomy only; this seems a reasonable approach when possible, especially when considering the biofilm theory of capsular contracture or retained foreign material (as in ruptured silicone gel devices) as causative for capsular contracture.

All the following may play a role in enhancing success.[25]

- Meticulous technique
- Precise hemostasis
- Conversion to a subpectoral plane
- Use of textured devices
- Ample washing with triple antibiotic solutions.

By the same token, the ideal type (human versus animal), thickness, size, or shape of ADM required to create the optimal effect has not been demonstrated. If ADM exerts its effects through stress shielding of myofibroblasts or a delay in the inflammatory response due to the slow repopulation of the matrix, it stands to reason that larger and thicker pieces might perform better than smaller and thinner ones.

After capsulectomy, the ADM may be inset anteriorly with interrupted or running absorbable sutures or fixed in place using parachute sutures that are exited through the skin, tied loosely, covered with an occlusive dressing and removed one week later. Drains are a necessity and are discontinued when the drainage is less than 20 ccs over a 24 hour period.

PATIENT EXAMPLES

Case 1

A 38-year-old patient who was 5 ft 8 in and 125 lbs underwent subpectoral augmentation with smooth-walled silicone gel devices and circumvertical mastopexy. At 1 year postoperatively, she developed a grade 3 capsular contracture of the right breast with high riding implant. At reoperation, a dense capsule was noted on the right. A total periprosthetic capsulectomy was performed; 6 × 16 cm piece of thick ADM was inset with running sutures to the anterior flap, and new implants were placed. Two years following revisionary surgery, a grade 1 capsule was present on the right (Case 1, **Figs. 1–4**).

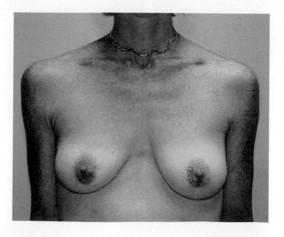

Fig. 1. Preoperative view.

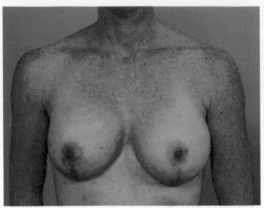

Fig. 2. 1.5 years postoperative subpectoral augmentation with smooth walled silicone gel implants and circumvertical mastopexy. Grade 3 capsular contracture right breast.

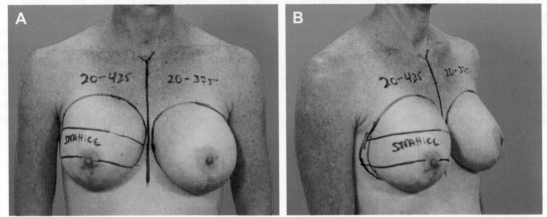

Fig. 3. (*A, B*) Operative plan: total periprosthetic capsulectomy and acellular dermal matrix placement; implant exchange.

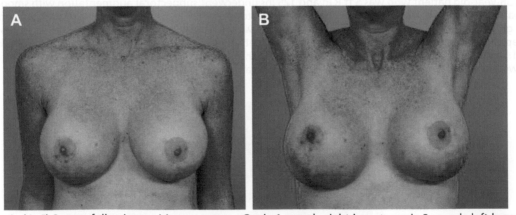

Fig. 4. (*A, B*) 2 years following revisionary surgery. Grade 1 capsule right breast; grade 2 capsule left breast.

Case 2: Capsular contracture

This case involved a 28-year-old, 5 ft 4 in, 115 lb patient. One year following subpectoral augmentation with smooth-walled silicone gel devices, she developed a grade 4 capsular contracture of left breast. At operation, a dense capsule was noted on the left; a total periprosthetic capsulectomy was performed and 4 × 16 cm pieces of thick ADM were placed bilaterally. Implants were exchanged. Grade 1 capsules are present bilaterally at 2 years (Case 2, **Figs. 5–8**).

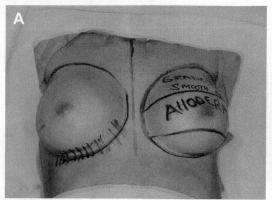 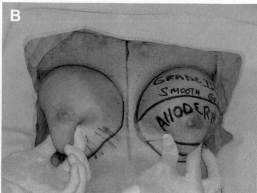

Fig. 5. (*A, B*) Intraoperative view: grade 4 capsular contracture left breast.

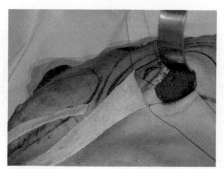

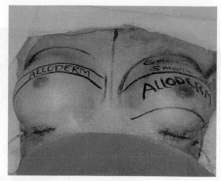

Fig. 6. Following total periprosthetic capsulectomy. Acellular dermal matrix draped over breasts and parachuted into position. Internal running sutures.

Fig. 7. Apperance at completion of revisionary surgery. Smooth implants exchanged for textured surface devices.

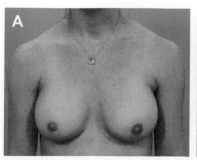 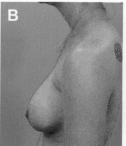 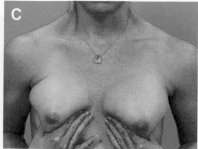

Fig. 8. (*A–C*) Appearance of breasts 2 years postoperatively. Grade 1 capsules bilaterally.

Case 3: Capsular contracture and poor tissue coverage

This case involved a 42-year-old patient with prior history of breast augmentation following bilateral nipple sparing mastectomies (right prophylactic, left breast cancer) and silicone gel implant reconstruction. She underwent postoperative radiation of the left breast. A grade 4 capsular contracture of left breast ensued with rippling and poor tissue coverage of the right breast. She desired smaller implants. Operative plan included near total capsulectomy of the right breast, with ADM placement (6 × 16 cm, thick), downsizing of implants bilaterally, conversion to textured devices, and ADM placement on the right to correct rippling. At 2 years postoperatively, grade 2 capsule is present on the left, and a grade 1 capsule is present on the right (Case 3, **Figs. 9–11**).

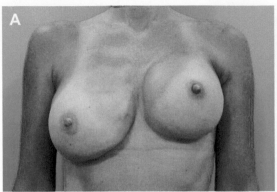 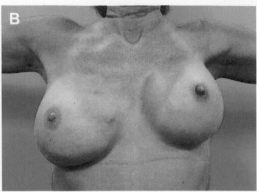

Fig. 9. (*A, B*) 42-year-old following bilateral nipple sparing mastectomies (right prophylactic, left breast cancer) and postoperative radiation of left breast. Grade 4 capsular contracture left breast. Rippling medially and thin coverage right breast.

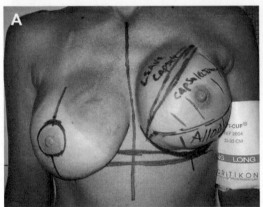 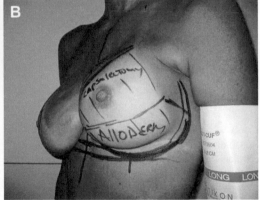

Fig. 10. (*A, B*) Before revisionary surgery. Plan near to total periprosthetic capsulectomies, acellular dermal matrix placement, pocket reshaping, implant exchange (downsize).

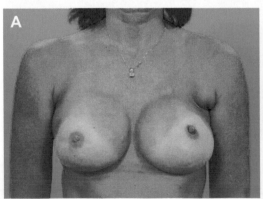 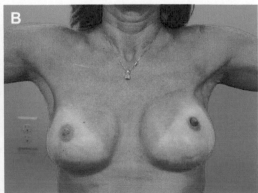

Fig. 11. (*A, B*) 2 years following revisionary surgery with acellular dermal matrix. Grade 2 capsule left; grade 1 capsule right.

Case 4: Ruptured saline device and capsular contracture

This case involved a 51-year-old, 5 ft 10 in 145 lb patient with pectus excavatum deformity. She underwent right breast augmentation subpectorally with a single silicone gel device in the 1970s. Subsequently, the patient had replacement with saline devices bilaterally in the 1990s. She presented with a ruptured saline device on the right right breast, and grade 3 capsular contracture of left breast. Intraoperative photos demonstrate planned placement of ADM and parachute sutures tied after devices were exchanged and drains placed. Fat was grafted to the upper pole of the right breast, and ADM was placed to correct step off (Case 4, **Figs. 12–16**).

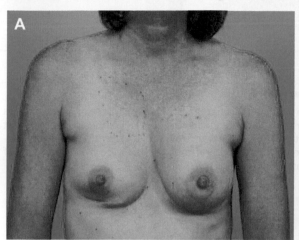
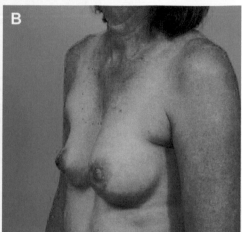

Fig. 12. (*A, B*) 51-year-old pectus deformity with deflation right saline breast implant and grade 3 capsular contracture left implant.

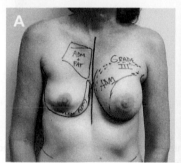
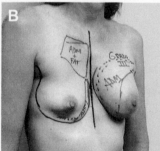
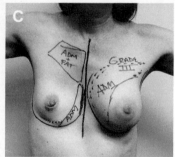

Fig. 13. (*A–C*) Before revisionary surgery. Plan total periprosthetic capsulectomies, acellular dermal matrix (ADM) placement left breast (breast plastic surgery [BPS] contour 2); ADM chest wall implant and fat grafting right upper chest step-off deformity. Bilateral implant exchange.

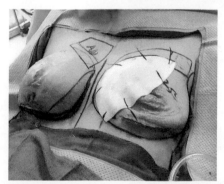
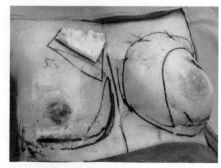

Fig. 14. Intraoperative view showing planned placement of acellular dermal matrix left.

Fig. 15. Intraoperative view stacked acellular dermal matrix for correction contour deformity upper right chest; parachute sutures exiting skin and tied loosely on left.

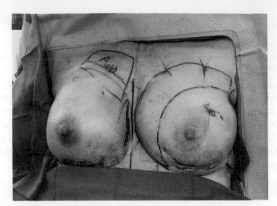

Fig. 16. At completion of revisionary surgery.

Case 5: Bilateral breast distortion with capsular contractures

This case involved a 67-year old 5 ft 3 in, 120 lb woman. This patient underwent bilateral mastectomies and reconstruction in the 1970s with expanders and silicone gel devices. She developed marked breast distortion bilaterally with grade 4 capsular contractures. Appearance 6 months after bilateral total peri-prosthetic capsulectomy, ADM placement (BPS contour 2), bilateral implant exchange with placement of textured wall devices, and fat grafting of breasts (Case 5, **Figs. 17–21**).

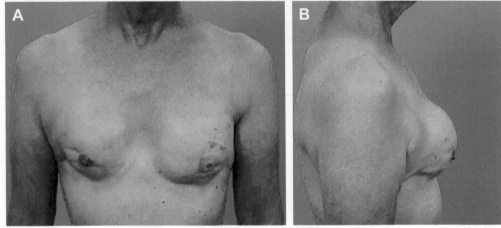

Fig. 17. (*A, B*) 67-year-old patient 30 years following bilateral mastectomies and expander/implant reconstruction. Profound distortion of breasts due to grade 4 capsular contractures.

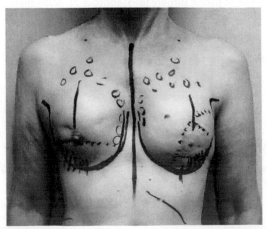

Fig. 18. Before revisionary surgery.

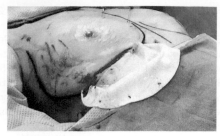

Fig. 19. Intraoperative view. Acellular dermal matrix (BPS contour 2) before inset with parachute sutures.

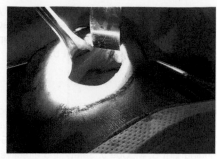

Fig. 20. Acellular dermal matrix inset into pocket.

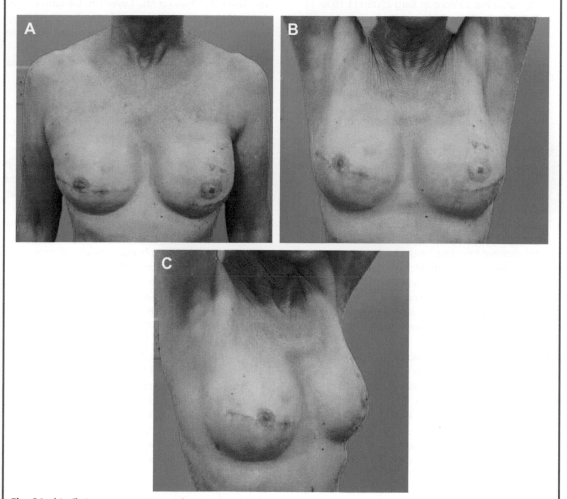

Fig. 21. (A–C) Appearance 6 months postoperatively.

SUMMARY

ADM for the prevention or correction of capsular contracture is effective in a variety of cases and appears to have a beneficial effect for up to 3 years. Adjunctive procedures for treating the capsule as well as the size, type, and thickness of the ADM required for optimal effectiveness have not been established. The longevity of correction has not been established. The mechanism by which ADM prevents or delays recurrent capsular contracture is at present unclear.

REFERENCES

1. Spear SL, Murphey DK, Slicton A, et al. Inamed silicone breast implant core study results at 6 years. Plast Reconstr Surg 2007;120(Suppl 1):S8–16.

2. Cunningham B, McCue J. Safety and effectiveness of Mentor's MemoryGel implants at 6 years. Aesthetic Plast Surg 2009;33:440–4.

3. Pajkos A, Deva AK, Vickery K, et al. Detection of subclinical infection in significant breast implant capsules. Plast Reconstr Surg 2003;111:1605–11.

4. El-Sheikh Y, Tutino R, Knight C, et al. Incidence of capsular contractufre in silicone versus saline cosmetic augmentation mamammoplasty: a meta-analysis. Can J Plast Surg 2008;16:211–5.

5. Wong CH, Samuel M, Tan BK, et al. Capsular contracture in subglandular breast augmentation with textured versus smooth breast implants: a systematic review. Plast Reconstr Surg 2006;118:1224–36.

6. Barnsley GP, SIgurdson LJ, Barnsley SE. Textured surface breast implants in the prevention of capsular contracture among breast augmentation patients: a meta-analysis of randomized controlled trials. Plast Reconstr Surg 2006;117:2182–90.

7. Gutkowski KA, Mesna GT, Cunningham B, et al. Saline filled breast implants: a plastic surgery educational foundation multicenter outcomes study. Plast Reconstr Surg 1997;100:1019–27.

8. Embrey M, Adams EE, Cuningham B, et al. A review of the literature on the etiology of capsular contracture and a pilot study to determine the outcome of capsular contracture interventions. Aesthetic Plast Surg 1999;23:197–206.

9. Holmich LR, Lipworth L, McLaughlin JK, et al. Breast implant rupture and connective tissue disease: a review of the literature. Plast Reconstr Surg 2007;120(Suppl 7):S62–9.

10. Cordiero PG, McCarthy CM. A single surgeon's 12-year experience with tissue-expander breast reconstruction: part II. An analysis of long-term complications, aesthetic outcomes and patient satisfaction. Plast Reconstr Surg 2006;118:832–9.

11. McCarthy CM, Pusic AL, Disa JJ, et al. Unilateral postoperative chest wall radiotherapy in bilateral expander/implant reconstruction patients: a prospective outcomes analysis. Plast Reconstr Surg 2005;116:1642–7.

12. Evans GR, Schusterman MA, Kroll S, et al. Reconstruction of the radiated breast: is there a role for implants? Plast Reconstr Surg 1995;96:1111–5.

13. Spear SL, Onyewu C. Staged breast reconstruction with saline-filled implants in the irradiated breast: recent rends and therapeutic implications. Plast Reconstr Surg 2000;105:930–42.

14. Kronowitz SL, Robb GL. Radiation and breast reconstruction: a critical review of the literature. Plast Reconstr Surg 2009;124:395–408.

15. Rudolph R, Abraham J, Vecchione T, et al. Myofibroblasts and free silicon around breast implants. Plast Reconstr Surg 1978;62:185.

16. Baker JL, Chandler ML, Levier RR. Occurrence and activity of myofibroblasts in human capsular tissue surrounding mammary implants. Plast Reconstr Surg 1981;68(6):905–12.

17. Hinz B. Formation and functiom of the myofibroblast during tissue repair. J Invest Dermatol 2007;127:526–37.

18. Katzel EB, Koltz PF, Tierney R, et al. The impact of Smad3 loss of function on TGF- β signaling and radiation-induced capsular contracture. Plast Reconstr Surg 2011;127(6):2263–9.

19. Zinman OA, Toblli J, Stella I, et al. The effects of angiotensin-converting enzyme inhibitors on the fibrous envelope around mammary implants. Plast Reconstr Surg 2007;120(7):2025–33.

20. Salzberg CA, Ashikari AY, Koch RM, et al. An 8-year experience of direct-to-implant immediate breast reconstruction using human acellular dermal matrix (AlloDerm). Plast Reconstr Surg 2011;127(2):514–37.

21. Maxwell GP, Gabriel A. Use of acellular dermal matrix in revisionary aesthetic breast surgery. Aesth Surg J 2009;29(6):485–93.

22. Stump A, Holton LH, Connor J, et al. The use of acellular dermal matrix to prevent capsule formation around implants in a primate model. Plast Reconstr Surg 2008;124(1):82–91.

23. Basu CB, Leong M, Hicks MJ. Acellular cadaveric dermis decreases the inflammatory response in capsule formation in reconstructive breast surgery. Plast Reconstr Surg 2010;126(6):1842–7.

24. Collis N, Sharpe DT. Recurrence of subglandular breast implant capsular contracture: anterior versus total capsulectomy. Plast Reconstr Surg 2000;106(4):792–7.

25. Adams WP Jr. Capsular contracture: what is it? What causes it? How can it be prevented and managed? Clin Plast Surg 2009;36(1):119–26.

Pocket Reinforcement Using Acellular Dermal Matrices in Revisionary Breast Augmentation

David Kaufman, MD

KEYWORDS

- Implant malposition • Bottoming out • Synmastia
- Lateral implant malposition • Implant problems • Asymmetry
- Acellular dermal matrix • Revisionary breast surgery

Key Points

1. The two most frequently encountered complications of primary breast augmentation are capsular contracture and implant malposition.

2. Each successive surgical revision is incrementally more challenging, thus each revision attempt must be planned thoroughly; understanding the anatomy of the primary augmentation failure is essential to properly diagnose and treat the unsatisfactory outcome.

3. Treatment of breast implant malposition depends largely on the patient's anatomy, presenting complaints, desired outcome, and anatomic limitations.

In 2010, close to 300,000 breast augmentations were performed in the United States, making this the most commonly performed cosmetic surgery.[1] By virtue of the sheer numbers of annual breast augmentations performed, a large market for revisionary augmentation procedures exists. The two most frequently encountered complications of primary breast augmentation are capsular contracture and implant malposition.[2] This article focuses on treatment of implant malposition, excluding capsular contracture, by using acellular dermal matrices (ADMs).

Implant malposition may occur in any one (or a combination) of the four breast quadrants.

1. Superior
2. Medial
3. Inferior
4. Lateral.

Superior displacement (high-riding implants) may result from inadequate pocket creation, insufficient release of the pectoralis major muscle, or secondarily as a presentation of capsular contracture (**Fig. 1**A).

Medial displacement (synmastia) is almost always an iatrogenic consequence resulting from overdissection of the pocket or selection of Implants that are too large.

Inferior displacement (bottoming out) is the most common malposition and presents as an elongation between the nipple areolar complex (NAC) and neoinframammary fold. This malposition may lead to stretching of the inferior breast pole skin, compromise of the integrity of the inframammary fold (IMF) structure, or a combination of the two (see **Fig. 1**B).

Lateral displacement of the implant is, to some degree, normal with submuscular implants, but excessive lateralization (telemastia) can create a wide separation between breasts (see **Fig. 1**C). Each of these deformities needs to be understood anatomically to institute proper revisionary surgery.

Disclosures: The author is a consultant for Mentor Corporation.
Kaufman and Clark Plastic Surgery, 2220 East Bidwell Street, Folsom, CA 95630, USA
E-mail address: David@thenaturalresult.com

Clin Plastic Surg 39 (2012) 137–148
doi:10.1016/j.cps.2012.02.001
0094-1298/12/$ – see front matter © 2012 Elsevier Inc. All rights reserved.

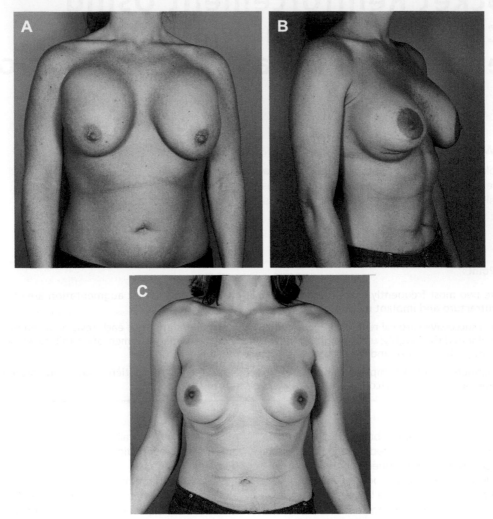

Fig. 1. (*A*) Implants high in relation to breast tissue. (*B*) Double-bubble deformity, in which the inframammary fold (IMF) has been violated. (*C*) Widely spaced implants as a consequence of a wide sternum and round rib cage.

ANATOMIC CONSIDERATIONS OF SECONDARY BREAST AUGMENTATION

Many challenges face the plastic surgeon when considering revisionary augmentation mammaplasty.[3] Patient dissatisfaction with the result of the initial procedure and secondary procedures creates unexpected costs and stress for patients who expected acceptable results with a single procedure. Each successive revision is incrementally more challenging, therefore it is crucial that each attempt at revision is done with as much forethought and planning as possible.

It is important to fully understand the anatomy of the primary augmentation failure to properly diagnose and treat the unsatisfactory outcome. Considerations include (**Table 1**):

- Nipple to sternal notch distance
- NAC to IMF distance
- Location of the current and original IMF
- Breast base width
- Potential presence of capsular contracture
- Plane location of the implants
- Approach location.

The following characteristics of the implants should be evaluated:

- Volume
- Surface texture
- Shape
- Type of implants.

When considering revision surgery, it is good practice to review the prior operative reports to

Table 1
Considerations for diagnosis and treatment of unsatisfactory outcomes

Measurement	Normal Dimension	Abnormality
Nipple to sternal notch	17–20 cm	Too long indicates the need for superior repositioning of the NAC
NAC to IMF	4–6 cm	Too long indicates the need for a mastopexy to reduce the bottom pole skin or repositioning of the IMF superiorly (for double-bubble deformity)
Location of IMF	Sixth rib	Too low indicates need to reposition the IMF
Base width	Variable	Assists with the selection of implants

learn as much as possible about the initial augmentation (or previous revisions) before undertaking further procedures.

PREVENTION OF DEFORMITY FOLLOWING PRIMARY AUGMENTATION

Before discussing treatment options and strategy for revision breast augmentation, it is important to understand how to prevent the unsatisfactory result. There are important anatomic considerations that the plastic surgeon must recognize and carefully manage during primary augmentation:

- Short NAC to IMF distance. In cases in which there is insufficient inferior breast pole skin, it is important to educate patients about the limitations this anatomic variation presents (**Fig. 2**A). After augmentation, the inferior pole expands, although it is typically not sufficient for the nipple to be positioned at the midportion of the breast mound. High-profile implants place the point of maximum projection lower on the breast and create more projection for the relative volume. It does this at the expense of sacrificing medial and upper pole fullness, although the trade-off usually leads to a better aesthetic result. Selection of modest-size implants is wise in these challenging cases, and although some surgeons are comfortable with lowering the IMF surgically, I find it perilous (see **Fig. 2**B).
- Round rib cage. A patient's skeletal anatomy has a significant role in the outcome of breast enhancement. Implants rest against the chest wall and their projection is perpendicular to a line tangent to the rib cage. Thus, women with round chests (see **Fig. 2**C) have implants that point radially outward, leading to a widened gap between the breasts and less projection of the implants. In this instance, patient education is again

crucial, because patients are more accepting of the outcome when this anatomic variation and its limitations are discussed beforehand. It is harder to satisfy a patient when this is explained after surgery. Wider-based implants are preferred in these patients because they create more medial fullness. Limiting lateral dissection, and even leaving a slip of pectoralis muscle laterally, can help with limiting the lateral shift of the implants.
- Long nipple to sternal notch distance. Many patients with long nipple to notch distances present seeking breast augmentation when they would benefit from a mastopexy. These patients (and some surgeons) think that placing large implants will fill the skin envelop adequately and avoid the increased scarring associated with breast lifting. It is crucial to have a frank discussion with patients who possess long nipple to notch distances, or nipples below the IMF, regarding the outcome without undergoing a breast lift. In these cases, some patients may achieve results that are satisfactory, although this is usually an exception. For borderline cases, sometimes a circumareolar mastopexy is considered. This approach may lead to early revision instead of a revolumized and lifted breast, because patients are left with larger, more droopy breasts. In addition, I have found that patients are uniformly disappointed by the poor cosmetic appearance of the resulting enlarged, distorted, and scarred areolas.
- Pectus excavatum. Just as round rib cages present challenges to the plastic surgeon, so too does pectus excavatum. Pectus excavatum results in a radially inward-oriented breast. In this instance, moderately sized implants are a better choice, because they lessen the kissing-breasts deformity.

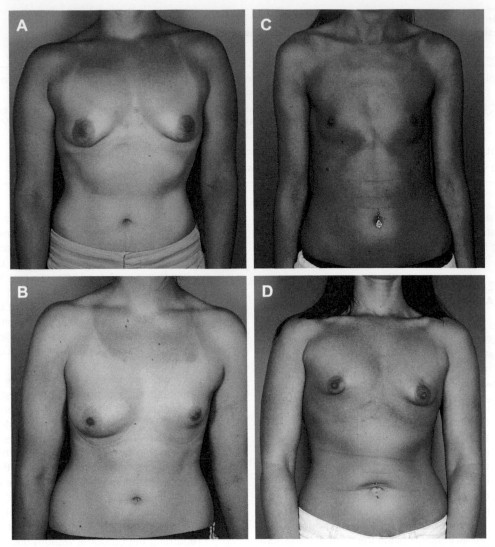

Fig. 2. (*A*) Short distance between NAC and IMF. (*B*) Marked volume asymmetry with vertical height difference between left and right IMF. (*C*) Round rib cage and widely spaced breasts. (*D*) Tuberous breast deformity with volume and IMF height asymmetry.

- Tuberous breasts, radiation damage, Poland syndrome, and severe asymmetry. Discussing each of these presentations is beyond the scope of this article, but recognition of the deformity, patient education, and creating the proper expectations of outcome are the keys to a satisfied patient (see **Fig. 2**D).

CURRENT TREATMENT OPTIONS WITHOUT THE USE OF ADM

Revision breast augmentation for deformity has a long history, although ADMs have only been in widespread use in plastic surgery during the last decade. The treatment of breast implant malposition depends largely on the patient's anatomy, presenting complaints, desired outcome, and anatomic limitations. This article reviews some of the tools available to help surgeons in the treatment of these deformities. The use of ADM is often complimentary.

- Plane exchange. Subglandular implants are prone to inferior displacement. There is little soft tissue for support and, as breast volume decreases, these implants are more likely to exhibit rippling and unacceptable palpability. Implants in the subglandular plane are also more susceptible to capsular contracture. Removal and replacement to a submuscular pocket may improve a great deal of the presenting complaints. It is debatable whether the prepectoral capsule needs to be removed. However, I find it is necessary to at least score the posterior wall, allowing the pectoralis muscle to expand. It is often necessary to use the inferior capsular wall to extend the reach of the pectoralis muscle and provide additional implant coverage in the lower outer quadrant.

- Capsular flaps. Following primary augmentation, especially in the setting of small breasts with large implants, there is often little soft tissue to work with during secondary procedures. Investigators have described using capsular flaps to reinforce pocket repair.[4] Although some have found success with these techniques, the use of capsular tissue cannot always be relied upon in the case of diseased capsule because the strength and longevity of capsular tissue are inconsistent.
- Muscle-splitting biplane. In cases of animation deformity, or subglandular bottoming out, a muscle-splitting biplane placement has been advocated.[2] This technique divides the pectoralis major muscle along its fibers and places the new implant in a partial subpectoral pocket. Superior pole coverage is provided and multiple-layer capsulorrhaphy is used to support the inferior and lateral implant pockets. A great deal of reliance is placed on the inferior capsulorrhaphy, and many investigators find that capsular repairs result in a high rates of recurrence.
- Capsulorrhaphy. Because there is often a paucity of manipulable tissue in the augmented breast, capsulorrhaphy remains a mainstay of revisionary strategy, especially in the setting of full or partially submuscular implants. Although capsular repair is generally technically easy, long-term results may be poor because the deforming forces that created the original deformity remain present and stretch the capsulorraphy, leading to recurrence.
- Neosubpectoral pockets. In the case of implants already in the submuscular plane, creation of a new submuscular pocket above the already present capsule provides the surgeon a fresh opportunity to create a better pocket for the implants. If the capsule is thin or wispy, it is technically challenging to keep the pockets separated.

- Fat grafting. Much interest has developed recently in fat grafting to the breast, and the topic of stem cells is often included in such discussions. There remains a great deal of confusion regarding the safety, efficacy, retention, and regenerative potential in this modality. Fat grafting is espoused by some to provide permanent volume augmentation, to reduce capsular contracture, and to smooth contour irregularities. However, all these are debated on many levels and additional studies are required to provide guidance for community practitioners.
- Mastopexy. If the nipple to notch distance is too long or there is too much inferior breast pole skin, a mastopexy is indicated to lift the nipple to the appropriate position on the breast mound or to redrape the skin as necessary. It is important to assess the implant position during these procedures because the implant can be bottomed out, the breast parenchyma may become ptotic, or both.

LESSONS LEARNED FROM THE USE OF ADM IN BREAST RECONSTRUCTION

During the last 10 years, ADMs have found widespread acceptance in breast reconstruction procedures, especially during immediate implant reconstruction. By extending the reach of the pectoralis major muscle, ADM allows for a greater degree of expander fill, which offers the advantages of reducing the initial deformity and maximizing the skin envelope. An excellent cosmetic outcome may be achieved because preserved mastectomy skin is optimized for reconstruction.[5] Expanders can be filled more rapidly, resulting in a shorter time from mastectomy to completion of reconstruction. The use of ADM may enable the creation of a submuscular pocket adequate to place a full-sized breast prosthesis, which allows maintenance of a fuller, thicker pectoralis muscle to cover the superior and medial implant poles.[6] The use of ADM can also improve soft tissue drapery around devices without resorting to the use of (nonpectoral) muscle or fascial flaps. Total device coverage with the use of combined ADM and pectoralis muscle coverage provides precise control of the pocket dimensions and permits more predictable aesthetic outcomes.[7]

CURRENTLY AVAILABLE ADM

ADM products were introduced to provide an additional tool for surgeons when faced with clinical scenarios in which autogenous tissues were inadequate. Currently, both human and animal sources are used to create allograft and xenograft ADM, respectively. Although each ADM manufacturer may have different techniques in processing the tissue, there is a common pathway.

Procuring Tissue

Tissue is procured through live or cadaveric donors or animal sources. The epidermal and subcutaneous layers are discarded during the initial procedure. All cells are removed, leaving only an acellularized dermis. The tissue is subsequently treated in either a disinfectant solution or irradiated, then cut to size and packaged (most ADMs are available in various thicknesses, sizes, and shapes). Differences between various ADMs can be seen in their production: some are lyophilized, some radiated, and some freeze dried. In addition, some products may need to be refrigerated and/or rehydrated.

Selection of ADM

The decision of which ADM to use is often a personal one, because many surgeons prefer a single product line and become comfortable with its performance. Cost is of concern, given that most patients seeking revisionary breast augmentation surgery have already incurred a high expense from the initial procedure, and the surgeon should be conscious of this stressor when offering revision options.[8] However, it has been my experience that most patients understand that revisions are more complex than primary surgery and each successive revision typically becomes more challenging. For the patient who has already undergone considerable psychological and financial stress from the unsatisfactory result of the initial operation, obtaining an optimal salvage through revision is of primary importance. Therefore, if the surgeon thinks that using a tool like ADM will make for the best outcome, patients will accept a higher cost.

I prefer Strattice™ (LifeCell Corporation, Branchburg, NJ, USA), derived from porcine tissue, for augmentation revision cases requiring ADM usage because of its predictable performance; specifically, the long-term resistance to stretch. This resistance allows accurate intraoperative visualization of the final result. There is some relaxation, but the repair tends to be robust and there is only a slight degree of repair stretch. In contrast, LifeCell's human cadaveric product Alloderm tends to relax and creates a greater misrepresentation

of the final result. In addition, the price of Strattice™ is among the lowest on the market.

TREATMENT OF INFERIOR AND/OR LATERAL IMPLANT DISPLACEMENT (BOTTOMING OUT) WITH ADM

The most common implant malposition is inferolateral displacement. Overdissection during primary implant placement and tissue atrophy over time are the primary causes. The challenge in correction of this deformity is the lack of good quality native tissue to support a repair. Capsular repair alone has a high degree of recurrence and can be unreliable because the capsule relaxes during the recovery period.

Author's Approach to ADM Placement

I have found that the use of ADM to reinforce the repair is an essential part of producing consistent and long-lasting results. Technically, the procedure I use is:

- Access the pocket and remove the current implant.
- Capsulotomies are performed as indicated.
- I then use a series of inverted 2-0 or 0 Vicryl sutures to repair the capsule and recreate the inferior and lateral borders of the pocket.
- Once this is done to my satisfaction, I place a sterile sizer in the pocket and fill it to the desired size.
- The patient is then sat upright to assess the new pocket configuration in various positions.
- These steps are repeated until I am satisfied with the symmetry and position of the breasts.
- The patient is returned to the supine position, the sizers are removed, and the pockets copiously irrigated with a gentamicin, bacitracin, and cefazolin solution.
- The ADM of choice is prepared as indicated, placed along the capsular border to reinforce the repair, and sutured into position. I place 10 to 12 sutures for each piece of ADM to ensure proper positioning. In addition, I also usually cut darts out of the ADM to allow it to curve along the shape of the implant without buckling.
- Next, a 10-French drain is placed between the ADM and the capsule to avoid seroma formation and to ensure adherence.
- The implants are then replaced and incisions closed in the usual fashion.

<table>
<tr><td>

Box 1
Key technical considerations in ADM in revision breast augmentation

1. Access pocket and remove implants
2. Perform capsulotomies/capsulectomies as necessary
3. Repair capsule or create inferior, lateral, and medial pocket borders
4. Reinforce with ADM as indicated
5. Drain
6. Irrigate, place implants, close
</td></tr>
</table>

Postprocedure Care for ADM Placement for Bottoming Out

- Early in the postoperative recovery phase, patients are placed into an underwire bra for support
- Drains are left in for between 3 and 7 days, depending on output
- During recovery it is important to limit heavy lifting or strenuous activity because the contraction of the pectoralis muscle can tear the capsular repair or disrupt the placement of the ADM
- I ask patients to avoid any pectoralis muscle activities for 2 months, such as push-ups or weight lifting exercises targeting the pectoralis muscles (**Box 1**).

The use of ADM can provide excellent results in cases of inferior (**Fig. 3**) and lateral displacement (**Figs. 4** and **5**).

TREATMENT OF MEDIAL IMPLANT DISPLACEMENT (SYNMASTIA) WITH ADM

Treatment of synmastia is particularly challenging. There are a variety of techniques described for repair and, as typically is the case when there are many techniques, none is definitively superior. The goal of synmastia repair is to separate the breast mounds and ensure that the tissue overlying the sternum remains immobile. If the implants are subglandular, then changing planes is usually necessary. If the implants are submuscular, changing to subglandular may be an option. However, I rarely place implants in the subglandular or subfascial space; in the short term, the revision may look acceptable, but my longer-term experience (>5 years) with subglandular implants has shown poor results.

I approach synmastia similarly to the correction of implant bottoming out:

- The implant pocket is accessed
- The implants are removed and the capsular work is performed
- I secure the medial capsule using sutures and evaluate the results of the capsuloplasty using sizers
- Once I am satisfied with the appearance of the temporary implants, I remove the sizers and secure an ADM sheet posteriorly before wrapping it around medially
- Parachute sutures are helpful to ensure that the medial breast skin stays adherent to the ADM
- A drain is placed and the procedure is completed in the same fashion as for

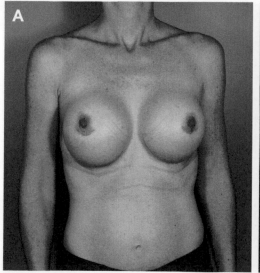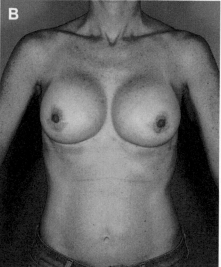

Fig. 3. (*A*) Implant malposition and asymmetry after placement of submuscular implants. (*B*) Result following pocket repair with lateral placement of ADM capsulorraphy.

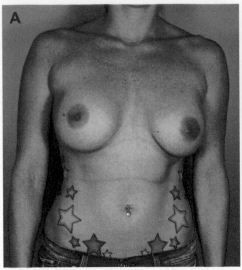
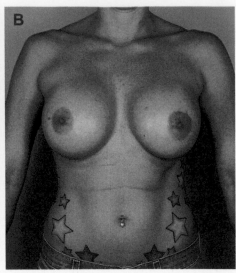

Fig. 4. (*A*) Lateral displacement of the left implant with resultant asymmetry. (*B*) After repair of capsule and repair of lateral and inferior capsule with ADM. A crescent lift was also concurrently performed on the left.

bottoming out (see section on the Author's Approach to ADM Placement).

POSTOPERATIVE CARE

When ADM products are used, the postoperative care is not significantly modified from the normal routine. The manufacturers of almost all ADM strongly suggest using drains around the ADM to reduce the rate of seroma formation.

- I typically use drains placed over the ADM to create a negative pressure seal between the overlying soft tissue and the ADM, and

with time the ADM will become vascularized. The thought process is similar to care of a skin graft, for which close apposition of the host tissue to graft is of paramount importance for graft take.

- I typically use an underwire bra as soon as the patient can tolerate it, because it provides an external bolster to the fold repairs. It is important to have the new pocket capsule form properly and symmetrically.
- Patients are urged not to lift anything more than 10 pounds for several weeks and to limit the use of chest wall musculature for 2 months.

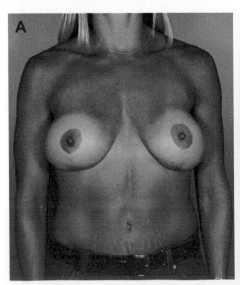
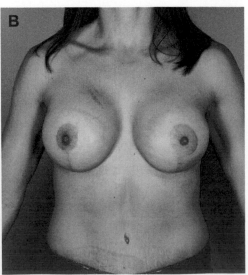

Fig. 5. (*A*) Lateral displacement of implants following mastopexy augmentation with submuscular implants. (*B*) After repair using larger implants and repair of lateral pocket with ADM.

Case study 1: Implant deformity

This 30-year old mother of 2 had submuscular 330-mL saline implants placed via a periareolar incision 7 years ago. She reported that her deformity was present shortly after surgery but, for various reasons, decided not to embark on early revision (**Fig. 6**A). Her presenting complaints included dissatisfaction with breast size, desire for increased cleavage, and inferolateral displacement of the implants. Options included upsizing, exchange to silicone gel implants, consideration of right-sided crescent mastopexy, and left implant repositioning with capsulorrhaphy and reinforcement with ADM. In addition, the placement of ADM on the left was considered to provide equal bilateral substrate so the tissues would age similarly.

Technical details:

- Under general anesthesia, the prior incisions were opened
- The capsules were opened and intact implants removed
- Superior and medial capsulotomies were performed as well as radial capsulotomies to accommodate a larger implant
- A series of 0 Vicryl inverted single interrupted sutures were used to perform the capsulorrhaphy
- A sterile sizer was placed to assess symmetry and assist in final implant selection
- Once symmetry was obtained, a 4 × 16 cm piece of Strattice™ was placed along each capsular repair to reinforce the new position of the lateral and inferior pocket
- The pockets were irrigated with triple-antibiotic solution and drains placed
- New 800-mL high-profile gel implants were placed and incisions closed
- The patient's NAC symmetry was assessed and a left circumareolar mastopexy was not performed

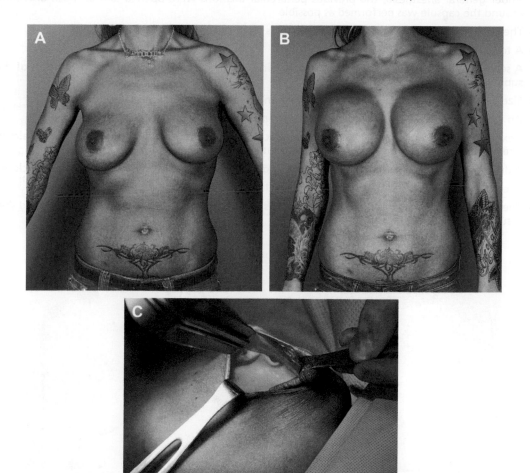

Fig. 6. (*A*) Unilateral bottoming out of the submuscular implant. Note the lack of superior pole and the elongated distance between the NAC and IMF. (*B*) After repair of capsule and placement of ADM. (*C*) Intraoperative photograph of the ADM placed to reinforce the lateral pocket.

Most patients are motivated to return to physical training regimens soon after surgery, but they are encouraged to do so with a modified routine. Exercise bicycles, treadmills, and ellipticals are all machines that can be used without invoking the pectoralis muscles. The concern is that, with contraction of the pectoralis muscles, pocket repairs may be disrupted and optimal results sacrificed. Patients understand these limitations and are typically compliant with the postoperative restrictions.

COMPLICATIONS WITH ADM

ADM is a foreign material, adding potential complications to consider. Two of the most common complications reported in the literature include infection and seroma.[9]

Infection Management

Infection is an uncommon sequela following placement of ADM. However, if signs of infection are present, such as redness, fevers, drainage, pain,

---

Case study 2: Bilateral implant malposition

This 43-year old woman presented 8 years after her third revision augmentation, with bilateral implant malposition, left Baker IV capsular contracture, severe asymmetry, and synmastia (**Fig. 7**A). She desired improved symmetry, treatment of her capsular contraction, slightly larger implants, and correction of synmastia.

Technical details:

- Under general anesthesia, the previous periareolar incisions were opened and as much dissection around the capsule was performed as possible
- The capsule was then opened and both implants were removed intact
- A total capsulectomy was then completed
- A series of Vicryl sutures were placed medially, inferiorly, and laterally to define the borders of the submuscular implant pockets
- Sizers were then placed to evaluate symmetry and the effect of the internal sutures
- An external bolster was placed to assist in creating a smooth arc along the pocket borders
- Next, a 4 × 16 cm piece of Strattice™ was placed along the medial and lateral pocket repairs to strengthen and reinforce the pocket-defining sutures
- A drain was placed and, after triple-antibiotic irrigation, the implants were placed and incisions closed
- The external bolsters and drains were removed 1 week after surgery
- The patient was placed into an underwire bra as soon as the external bolster was discontinued (her results are shown at 4 months; see **Fig. 7**B)

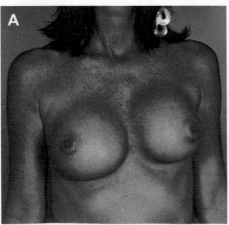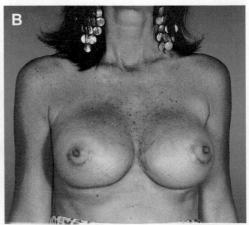

Fig. 7. (*A*) Right medial implant displacement, left capsular contraction, and implant malposition following breast augmentation and 2 revision procedures. (*B*) Result after capsulectomy, pocket repair, and reinforcement with ADM.

or swelling, management is often a challenge. The conventional wisdom is to expeditiously remove both the ADM and implant. Then, after eradication of infection with antibiotics and time to soften the surrounding tissue, patients are advised to return in 6 months for replacement of the implants.

In my experience, most patients resist accepting the necessity of implant removal. Occasional success can be achieved with removal of the implants, copious irrigation, and removal of all ADM, and then replacement with new implants in a single operation. However, this is often a costly

misadventure and caution is urged if this approach is undertaken.

Seroma

In normal circumstances, seromas are benign complications. However, the problem is more complex when using ADM. If a seroma forms around an ADM, it often leads to encapsulation of the graft instead of the normal course of integration and vascularization. If the ADM becomes encapsulated, it can not optimally perform its

---

Case study 3: Breast augmentation dissatisfaction

This 32-year old woman presented with generalized dissatisfaction following breast augmentation several years ago (**Fig. 8**A). She thought that her implants were too far apart, too small, and that her breasts were not attractive.

Technical details:

- Her procedure involved opening the previous inframammary incisions and capsules. Each capsule was thin and wispy.

- The implants were removed and a capsulotomy medially and superiorly was performed, thereby allowing a larger pocket to be created for the new implants to be repositioned superiorly and medially.

- A lateral capsuloplasty was performed to close the inferolateral pocket.

- Sizers were used to ensure that the pocket was properly modified and the results would be consistent with the patient's desires.

- A drain was placed.

- ADM was sutured in place inferiorly and laterally for pocket reinforcement.

- Silicone memory gel implants were placed and the incisions closed.

Postoperative photographs are shown at 6 months (see **Fig. 8**B).

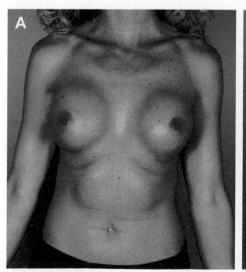 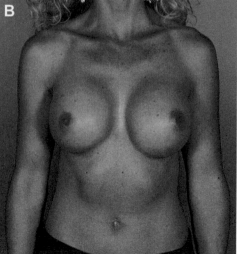

Fig. 8. (*A*) Lateral displacement of implants after submuscular placement via IMF approach. (*B*) Result following upsizing and lateral pocket repair with placement of ADM.

reinforcing function. In addition, a seroma around the ADM increases the probability of infection. When a seroma is present, placement of a seroma catheter drain can adequately treat the problem, but establishing the diagnosis is a challenge. Instead, I have found that placing a drain during surgery, so that it rests on top of the ADM, and leaving it in place for 5 days has eliminated problems with seroma formation.

ADM FOR REVISION BREAST AUGMENTATION: SUMMARY

ADM products have been shown to be an invaluable resource in revisionary breast augmentation procedures, validated both in the plastic surgery literature as well as in my own experience.[8,10,11] It is an ideal soft tissue substitute because of the lack of antigenicity and its ability to become integrated and vascularized into the host. These biologic materials also provide the intraoperative benefit of accurate long-term visualization of results, because ADM are generally resistant to stretch over time (some products more than others). In addition, the material provides strength and consistency that I think are superior to a patient's native tissue (such as capsular flaps) in providing reliable reinforcement for new implant pocket creation. Although high cost may be a drawback, the overall benefit is worth it because patients can be more assured of a reliable and aesthetically pleasing revision that is preferable to the psychological and financial stress of further revisions. I urge all plastic surgeons to consider this tool in their cosmetic and reconstructive breast practice.

REFERENCES

1. American Society of Plastic Surgeons. "2010 cosmetic surgery statistics." Available at: http://www.plastic surgery.org/Documents/news-resources/statistics/2010-statisticss/Overall-Trends/2010-cosmetic-plastic-surgery-minimally-invasive-statistics.pdf. Accessed August 25, 2011.

2. Khan UD. Combining muscle-splitting biplane with multilayer capsulorrhaphy for the correction of bottoming down following subglandular augmentation. Eur J Plast Surg 2010;33:259–69.

3. Adams WP, Teitelbaum S, Bengston BP, et al. Breast augmentation roundtable. Plast Reconstr Surg 2006;118(Suppl 7):175S–87S.

4. Voice SD, Carlsen LN. Using a capsular flap to correct breast implant malposition. Aesthet Surg J 2001;21:441–4.

5. Sbitany H, Sandeen S, Amalfi A, et al. Acellular dermis-assisted prosthetic breast reconstruction versus complete submuscular coverage: a head-to-head comparison of outcomes. Plast Reconstr Surg 2009;124(6):1735–40.

6. Zienowicz R, Karacaoglu E. Implant-based breast reconstruction with allograft. Plast Reconstr Surg 2007;120:373–81.

7. Namnoum J. Expander/implant reconstruction with Alloderm: recent experience. Plast Reconstr Surg 2009;124:387–94.

8. Hartzell T, Taghinia AH, Chang J, et al. The use of human acellular dermal matrix for the correction of secondary deformities after breast augmentation: results and cost. Plast Reconstr Surg 2010;126(5):1711–20.

9. Newman M, Swartz KA, Samson MC, et al. The true incidence of near term postoperative complications in prosthetic breast reconstruction utilizing human acellular dermal matrices: a meta-analysis. Aesthetic Plast Surg 2011;35:100–6.

10. Maxwell G, Gabriel A. Use of the acellular dermal matrix in revisionary aesthetic breast surgery. Aesthet Surg J 2009;29:485–93.

11. Spear S, Seruya M, Clemens MW, et al. Acellular dermal matrix for the treatment and prevention of implant-associated breast deformities. Plast Reconstr Surg 2011;127:1047.

The Use of Human Acellular Dermal Matrices in Irradiated Breast Reconstruction

Bruce M. Topol, MD

KEYWORDS

- Breast reconstruction • Radiation • Acellular dermal matrix
- Tissue expander • Fat graft • Implant capsule

Key Points: ACELLULAR DERMAL MATRICES RADIATION BREAST RECONSTRUCTION

1. External beam radiation has acute and chronic deleterious effects on wound healing in breast reconstruction, and thus the quality of the reconstruction itself.

2. Complication rates of 30% to 60% were reported following radiation to an implant breast reconstruction before the use of acellular dermal matrices (ADM) materials.

3. Complication rates for irradiated implant reconstructions have been lowered with the use of ADM materials, but the quality of the irradiated reconstruction is likely inferior to nonirradiated reconstruction.

4. A staged approach to the irradiated implant reconstruction is advised, which involves placement of a tissue expander followed later by implant exchange.

5. It is helpful, at the stage of initial tissue expander reconstruction, to:
   - Secure the ADM material to the overlying breast skin flap with internal quilting sutures
   - Secure the intramammary fold with permanent sutures

6. The irradiated breast implant reconstruction can be improved with additional pieces of ADM material, capsulectomy, and fat grafting at the time of expander removal/implant exchange. Fat grafting can be done at a later stage.

Roentgen discovered the x-ray in 1895.[1] Within 1 year, Gocht in Germany treated the first 2 patients with x-ray radiation for painful locally advanced disease and obtained relief,[2] demonstrating the potential benefits of radiation. Shortly thereafter, in 1901, Becquerel noted the deleterious effects of radiation when he reported that he developed a wound on his chest skin after leaving a vial of radium in his breast pocket for 6 hours. He noted the acute erythema and subsequent ulceration that took a prolonged time to heal.[1] Thus, the double-edged sword that is radiation became known to physicians, and this therapeutic/wounding effect has remained a challenge to this day.

IONIZING RADIATION

Energy from radiation can be absorbed by biological material and can result in excitation of electrons in the tissue or ionization of the atoms within this tissue. Release of enough ionizing energy within the tissue can cause localized

---

There are no financial interests or disclosures.
Division of Plastic Surgery, The Elliot Hospital, Catholic Medical Center, 36 Bay Street, Manchester, NH 03104, USA
E-mail address: drtopol@drtopol.com

Clin Plastic Surg 39 (2012) 149–158
doi:10.1016/j.cps.2012.02.002

damage to that tissue. This damage, known to medicine for longer than a century, can be therapeutic or harmful depending on several factors.

Radiation can be classified as electromagnetic or particulate. Electromagnetic radiation such as the short-wavelength x-ray can cause damage to human tissue, as can the particulate radiation produced by discrete particles such as electrons and protons (among others). This particulate radiation can be delivered by a variety of techniques, by intracavitary means or via external beam. This article discusses the effects of external beam radiation therapy in common use today, but recognizes that newer techniques of intracavitary and partial breast irradiation are currently being evaluated.[3]

EXTERNAL BEAM RADIATION

As would be expected, the higher the beam energy, the deeper the penetration into human tissue. Earlier beam energy devices were relatively lower-voltage x-ray machines that delivered low energy and were only able to penetrate superficially into tissue. These devices are termed orthovoltage, and are still useful for skin irradiation. Most breast tumors are now treated with high-energy megavoltage machines, commonly a linear accelerator, which can generate beams of sufficient energy to penetrate deeper into tissue.

The unit of measure of the biological effect in tissue caused by radiation is termed the radiation absorbed dose or rad. At present the gray (Gy) is used to represent 100 rad. Thus the more commonly used 50 Gy is equivalent to 5000 rad.

The degree of tissue penetration for a given radiation dose varies depending on the energy delivered. Fortunately, depth of penetration can be calculated very precisely for the different energy sources, and this depth of maximum dose (D_{max}) follows a predictable curve. Initially there is a zone of superficial penetration with a rapid buildup of energy, then a loss of energy as the beam penetrates deeper in the case of low-energy orthovoltage radiation. This process would yield the greatest effect in the skin, for example. By contrast, the high-energy megavoltage beam would have a slow buildup of energy superficially and reach its maximal energy deeper in the tissue, thus sparing the skin from the maximal radiation effect and damage while delivering the maximal effect and damage to tumors deeper in the tissue, such as the breast.

DOSING SCHEDULE FOR RADIATION

The fact that certain cells are more sensitive to the effects of radiation than others was first noted in

1906.[1] Since then it has become clear that cells are most sensitive to the effects of radiation during the G2-M phase of the cell cycle and are most resistant during the S phase.[1] Thus, a single dose of radiation will not affect all the cells that are irradiated, because of differences in cell-cycle status. This situation has led to the concept of fractionation or delivery of radiation in installments over time, which is the current practice.

RADIATION EFFECTS ON SKIN AND WOUND HEALING

As noted earlier, the effect of radiation on skin has been known for more than a century. Radiation has both acute and chronic effects that, of course, vary with the type, dose, and delivery schedule used.[1,4]

The acute effects include erythema, dry desquamation at lower doses, and moist desquamation at higher doses. The erythema is the direct result of an inflammatory process caused by increased capillary permeability. Dry desquamation is the result of a dose of radiation strong enough to kill some epidermal cells, but allowing enough of the remaining epidermal cells to survive and proliferate. Moist desquamation occurs when an inadequate number of epidermal cells survive and the exposed dermis oozes serous fluid.

The chronic effects include either an increase or a decrease in pigmentation, thickening and fibrosis of the skin, telangiectasia, and alteration of hair, sweat, and sebaceous gland function. Pigmentation is altered by death of melanocytes or by deposition of pigment into the dermis. Dermal thickening can occur, as the collagen within the involved dermis will swell. If the dose is strong enough, fibroblasts are impaired and unable to synthesize collagen, and the dermis will atrophy and could ulcerate. Telangiectasia is the result of thrombosis of deeper vessels. Active hair follicles and sebaceous glands are killed by the radiation. This aspect is particularly important, because these structures provide migrating epidermal cells that are necessary for reepithelialization and wound repair.

As a direct result of these effects, a skin wound that is radiated is prone to prolonged healing, with a resultant scar that is thin in the dermis as well as the epidermis, has poor vascularity and strength, is susceptible to opening, and is unable to defend adequately against infection.

EFFECTS OF RADIATION ON EXPANDED SKIN IN THE ANIMAL MODEL

Understanding the effects of radiation on skin, soft tissue, and wound healing, the question occurs as to what effects radiation may have on expander/ implant (silicone or saline) breast reconstruction. A few studies have examined the effects of radiation on previously expanded skin in an animal model. Goodman and colleagues[5] used New Zealand white rabbits and evaluated the effects of radiation on expanded skin 6 weeks after a single radiation dose of 25 to 35 Gy. A thickening of the epidermis but no change to the dermis was found, although the histology was performed only 6 weeks postradiation. Dvali and colleagues[6] studied effects of radiation on Yorkshire pigs. Skin was irradiated in fractions up to a total dose of 48.6 Gy and expanders placed under this skin 3 months later, and the skin flaps were then expanded. The skin flaps were evaluated almost 6 months after completion of the radiation. At this time the irradiated skin flaps were reduced in overall area by 23% compared with nonirradiated controls. It was also found that radiation reduced expanded skin flap viability by almost one-third compared with controls. Performing a capsulectomy did not significantly worsen this decreased viability.

EFFECTS OF RADIATION ON PROSTHETIC BREAST RECONSTRUCTION BEFORE THE USE OF ACELLULAR DERMAL MATRICES

Much has been written on the effects of radiation on silicone and saline implant breast reconstruction. It is helpful to review the literature published before the introduction of acellular dermal matrices (ADM) in these reconstructions, to better assess the effects of the radiation with the subsequent use of these materials and to determine if there are any differences.

Given the proven negative effects of radiation on wound healing, it is not surprising that external beam radiation has been shown to exert a negative effect on the outcome of breast reconstruction using tissue expanders and saline or silicone implants.

Krueger and colleagues[7] showed a 68% complication rate for tissue expander/implant reconstructions that were irradiated postoperatively compared with a 31% complication rate without radiation, resulting in a reconstructive failure rate of 37% compared with an 8% failure rate without radiation. Other reports show very high complication rates, high Baker III-IV capsule rates, and higher rates of reconstructive failure resulting in expander or implant loss when radiation follows tissue expander/implant reconstructions.[8–11]

Similarly, Spear and Onyewu[12] reported on a variety of tissue expander/implant reconstructions treated with and without radiation, and included reconstructions that had been irradiated

before reconstruction, during expansion, and after reconstruction. A capsular contracture rate of 32.5% was found, regardless of when the patient received the radiation, compared with a rate of zero in the nonirradiated group. There was also a 37.5% incidence of adding a transverse rectus abdominis muscle (TRAM) or latissimus flap in the radiated group versus a 10% incidence in the nonirradiated patients to either salvage or improve the cosmesis of the reconstruction. Indeed, to combat these very high rates of complications, advanced capsule formation, and/or implant loss, Spear and Onyewu advise their patients that addition of a TRAM or latissimus flap at the time of expander removal/implant exchange will be needed in 50% of cases involving radiation.

Parsa and colleagues[13] advise delaying reconstruction by at least 6 months after radiation to assess skin damage, and then to proceed with expander/implant reconstruction if there is no induration and moderate or better skin changes.

Kronowitz and colleagues[14] propose a delayed-immediate reconstruction whereby an expander is placed immediately at the time of the mastectomy and, if radiation is needed postoperatively, the expander is left in place until completion of the radiation, before being replaced by an autologous flap.

Fine and Hirsch[15] at Northwestern suggest a similar plan, but do not routinely place an autologous flap after radiation, and use an implant depending on desires of the patient.

Cordeiro and colleagues[16] reported a totally different timetable whereby the tissue expander is placed immediately and inflated during subsequent chemotherapy, then replaced with an implant before initiation of radiation therapy. These investigators report very similar results between the irradiated and nonirradiated groups overall in terms of complications, with only a higher Baker III capsule rate among the irradiated reconstructions.

Despite these various protocols, tissue expansion followed by implant/exchange breast reconstruction continues to challenge us all as plastic surgeons, especially when the reconstruction has been or will be irradiated. The question is what effect, if any, has ADM had on these problems? To answer this question one needs to briefly examine the relatively short history of ADM and implant breast reconstruction, which is examined in greater detail in the article by Baxter elsewhere in this issue.

BRIEF REVIEW OF ADM AND IMPLANT RECONSTRUCTION

Although the use of ADM in immediate breast reconstruction is relatively new, first reported in

2001,[17] its use has dramatically increased in popularity since then. Many publications support its use, safety, and efficacy in immediate single-stage implant (silicone, saline, adjustable) reconstruction[17–21] as well as in a 2-stage tissue expander/implant exchange technique.[22,23] The use and history of these materials is well covered elsewhere in this issue and is not the focus of this article. Previous work has shown histologically that human dermal allograft promotes less fibrosis and inflammation in capsules formed around implants.[24] The history and the expanding use of these materials is, however, important in evaluating these materials in the context of breast irradiation. As experience with these materials has increased, so have the applications that are generating more reports and evaluations of ADM materials subjected to radiation during the course of breast reconstruction.

EXPERIMENTAL EVIDENCE FOR PROTECTIVE EFFECT OF ADM IN IRRADIATED PROSTHETIC RECONSTRUCTION

In an important animal study, Komorowska-Timek and colleagues[25] reported on the protective effect of AlloDerm®. (LifeCell Corp, Branchburg, NJ, USA), a popular human acellular dermal matrix, on irradiated implant capsules formed in Sprague-Dawley rats using small saline implants. The implants were inflated and irradiated 2 days later with a single dose of 21.5 Gy. The resultant capsules were examined at 3 weeks postradiation and a second group at 12 weeks postradiation, and compared with irradiated non-AlloDerm® controls and nonirradiated controls. The AlloDerm® group was seen to have a protective effect on the radiation changes that were seen. There was less radiation-related inflammation and, importantly, only 1 of the 20 rats that were radiated developed a pseudoepithelium on the AlloDerm®, whereas all of the non-AlloDerm® radiated control capsules developed this pseudoepithelium. These findings, which have been confirmed elsewhere,[26] are very important because it is believed that formation of this pseudoepithelium is a precursor to the formation of a fibrotic capsule in humans.[27]

Armed with the knowledge of the protective effects of ADM on irradiated implant capsules in the animal model and knowing that ADM has been shown to diminish inflammation and fibrosis in capsules formed around implants in humans, the question is whether ADM offers any protective benefit to an implant breast reconstruction that has been or will be radiated. An increasing body of literature has evaluated the results of implant breast reconstruction using ADM that have been

radiated. Less has been written on the effects of radiation if the radiation has preceded the reconstruction.

EFFECTS OF RADIATION ON ADM/TISSUE EXPANDER OR IMPLANT BREAST RECONSTRUCTIONS

In an elegant review of 12 published studies on complication rates in prosthetic breast reconstruction using ADM, Newman and colleagues[28] found an overall complication rate of 12%.

More recently, Salzberg and colleagues[17] reported a complication rate of 3.9% following an 8-year experience using ADM and immediate implant reconstruction. Their review reported a 14.3% complication rate if the reconstruction was irradiated (this included either prereconstruction or postreconstruction radiation) which, though greater than their complication rate without radiation, is still consistent with the 12% reported by Newman in the absence of radiation.

Further evaluation by Nahabedian[29] reviewed the rate of infection, seroma, and skin necrosis in prosthetic reconstructions using AlloDerm® both with and without radiation. Nahabedian found that the timing of the radiation (prereconstruction or postreconstruction) was not a factor. He also found an infection rate of 3.9% without radiation and 9.4% with either preoperative or postoperative radiation. Seromas occurred in 2.6% of nonirradiated breasts and in 13% of irradiated breasts. No irradiated breast showed skin necrosis. Wound dehiscence occurred in 1.3% of nonirradiated breasts and in 13% of irradiated breasts. Statistical significance of these differences was not evaluated; the number of all these complications was small.

In a review of 231 patients undergoing a 2-stage prosthetic reconstruction, Seruya and colleagues[30] found a 15.4% capsule rate in irradiated reconstructions versus 2% in nonirradiated reconstructions, but no difference in the revision rate or the rate of explantation caused by infection after stage 2.

Again, it is important that even though the effects of radiation increased the number of complications even with ADM, this increased rate is still consistent with the overall rate noted by Newman and colleagues[28] in their meta-analysis of complications in nonirradiated reconstructions. Perhaps most importantly, the complication rates in prosthetic reconstructions using ADM discussed here are markedly less than the greater than the 40% complication rates described by Christante and colleagues[8] and also by Ascherman and colleagues[11] when ADM was not used with the prosthetic reconstruction that was irradiated.

THE USE OF FAT GRAFT IN RADIATED TISSUE

The newest addition to prosthetic breast reconstruction involves the use of fat grafting. After pioneering work by Coleman,[31] the use of staged, serial fat grafts as an adjunct to fill and soften implant reconstructions has been shown to be very effective even in the face of radiation.[32,33] The fat is injected after completion of the radiation either at the time of delayed insertion of a tissue expander, at the time of implant exchange, or subsequent to implant exchange and the demarcation of deformity around the implant.

THE AUTHOR'S APPROACH TO IRRADIATED BREAST RECONSTRUCTION

Like many approaches to problems in plastic surgery, a staged approach is appropriate when dealing with the prosthetic breast reconstruction that has been or will be irradiated. My approach varies depending on the quality of the tissue at the time of the reconstruction. I find it is the quality of the skin/soft tissue that is most important and that the occurrence of the radiation (prereconstruction or postreconstruction) carries less of an impact. Working with a hard reconstruction under skin that is heavily pigmented and telangiectatic from radiation 10 years previously can be less satisfying than with a breast reconstruction that was irradiated after tissue expander placement 3 or 4 months previously that is relatively soft and minimally pigmented.

To begin with, I believe it is better to perform implant reconstructions in 2 stages, for 3 reasons:

1. I believe a partially inflated tissue expander causes less tension on the overlying wound and soft tissue than a fully "inflated" implant.
2. It has also been my observation (I do not yet have objective data) that the thicker shell of a tissue expander is subject to less deformation than the thinner shell of an implant when subjected to radiation; I think it holds its shape better.
3. Planning ahead of time that we will be "going back" allows me to perform adjunct work on the capsule, adjust implant borders, and place additional ADM and/or fat graft if necessary without having to convince the reluctant patient who feels the reconstruction is "good enough" when I know it can be much better.

I also prefer to do opposite breast symmetry work at the time of the second stage when I have a much clearer idea of what the unilateral reconstruction looks like.

The vast majority of my reconstructions are immediate. I do not always know if radiation will or will not be used when I am in the operating room. I follow the same protocol regardless. I have used many different types of ADM, all with similar good results. I currently use AlloDerm® (LifeCell Corp, Branchburg, NJ, USA). I rarely see the "red breast" on the overlying skin flap but when I do, I worry and treat with oral antibiotics, although it is likely due to inflammation rather than infection. I will gladly switch to a different product when one becomes less expensive than what is currently available, provided continued reliability is consistent with what I use now.

THE AUTHOR'S OPERATIVE TECHNIQUE FOR PLACING THE ADM

When the mastectomy incision is in the mid-breast at the nipple areola (either excising or sparing it):

- I suture the inferior edge of the ADM to the inferior breast skin flap from a point approximately 1 cm above the inframammary fold (IMF) from medial to lateral and then continue up and around the lateral mammary fold to the lateral upper border of the elevated pectoralis muscle.
- I then suture the ADM to the inferior skin flap with several 3-0 absorbable sutures in an internal quilting fashion variously at the mid-height of the ADM and up to the upper one-quarter of the flap height.
- If available, I select a piece of ADM with a height equal to the height of the skin from the IMF to the incision. In this way I have good opposition of the ADM to the overlying skin flap and no drain is needed in this location. This action also will minimize any downward pull of the muscle by too short a piece of ADM, which can exacerbate the skin envelope shape difference between the operated and the opposite breast.
- I use permanent 2-0 polyester suture in an interrupted fashion to secure the IMF and lateral fold to the chest wall fascia/muscle to reconstruct the borders of the breast pocket, which have usually been violated by the mastectomy. I believe this helps reduce the typical elevation of the IMF that occurs with radiation, and prevents lateral displacement of the device (**Fig. 1**). I warn patients in advance that these are the sutures that hurt after the surgery,

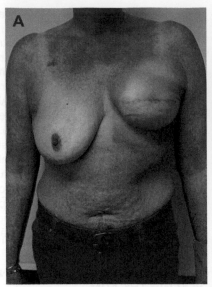 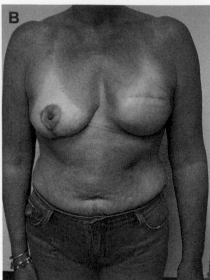

Fig. 1. (*A*) Typical elevation of implant and inframammary fold (IMF) after radiation. (*B*) Postoperative appearance after lowering the left IMF only, and a vertical mastopexy on the right.

especially the lateral sutures into the serratus muscle.

- I place a #7F drain through a long subcutaneous tunnel to drain the pocket and device. I do not usually place a drain over the muscle/under the upper skin flap.
- If an axillary dissection has been done, I drain the axilla but try to cover the drain with lateral soft tissue to separate the axilla and this drain from the breast wound, as I may need to leave the axillary drain in longer than the breast pocket drain.
- Once the tissue expander is placed, I suture the superior margin of the ADM to the inferior margin of the muscle with interrupted figure-of-8 2-0 absorbable sutures. It is important to make sure that this suture line is below or inferior to the skin incision so that if the wound opens, exposed muscle will be seen rather than exposed ADM that may not yet be revascularized.
- Before complete closure I place a 21-gauge butterfly needle under direct vision through the skin/muscle into the expander fill dome. Filling proceeds to a point about one-half to two-thirds of the breast volume as measured by the weight of the mastectomy specimen in the operating room.
- The wound is closed in layers and dressed.
- I use a BioPatch (Ethicon, Somerville, NJ, USA) at the drain exit site, as it is a chlorhexidine impregnated dressing with a central hole that allows passage of the drain tube through it, to minimize bacterial ingress along the drain tract into the expander cavity.

- This dressing is covered with 2 layers of clear plastic dressing. I have found this dressing can be left in place for 2 weeks without any evidence of skin irritation at the drain insertion site.
- If the mastectomy incision is in the IMF then the superior margin of the ADM is sutured to the inferior margin of the muscle first, followed by the quilting sutures, followed by the permanent pocket sutures, before placing the drain and closing the wound.

Postoperative Care

- A surgical bra is placed, and patients are typically discharged from hospital the next morning, even in bilateral cases.
- I continue oral antibiotics for 1 week and remove the drain(s) when output is less than 50 mL in 24 hours.
- Irradiated patients, obese fatty breasts, and axillary dissection patients drain longer.
- I get anxious if significant drainage persists for longer than 14 days, and I may pull the drain. Occasionally this results in the need for percutaneous aspiration with ultrasound guidance/protection.

THE AUTHOR'S ALGORITHM FOR THE EXPANDER/IMPLANT EXCHANGE

The decision as to what to do, and when, after radiation depends on the appearance and quality of the skin/soft tissue over the tissue expander. Where I work, the radiation oncologists prefer that I do not fully inflate the expander before radiation.

Once the radiation course has been completed, I begin to consider the implant exchange no sooner than 3 months after radiation. I believe the skin is too acutely damaged before this time. When the skin is not heavily pigmented and not indurated, I plan the exchange procedure. This procedure may be at the 3-month point or could be delayed for 9 months or so if the radiation was given postoperatively. If the radiation was given more than 1 year ago (as would be the case with a completion mastectomy following a recurrence after lumpectomy/radiation done in the past), the second stage can commence as early as 6 weeks after placing the expander, depending on skin quality. When I determine that the skin/soft tissue is optimal for that patient, I use an algorithm for the second-stage procedure(s). I use the same algorithm if I am working on a reconstruction that was done in one stage with an implant at the time of the reconstruction (**Fig. 2**).

The second-stage procedure is straightforward expander removal and implant exchange. I advise smooth round silicone gel implants (I do not have access to the shaped, highly cohesive gel implants). Implant size is based on patient preference for size (often larger, rarely smaller), skin envelope quality, base diameter of the breast pocket, and the size and shape of the opposite breast in unilateral cases. It is important to fill the base diameter to minimize lateral shift and cleavage widening. I place an implant that is larger in volume than the expander because I believe the volume of the expander shell is 50 to 100 mL greater than the shell of the implant, and this must be accounted for.

This straightforward exchange is easiest but, in my practice, not a common situation.

Non-Straightforward Implant Exchange Procedure

Frequently the capsule is firm and implant exchange must be accompanied by anterior capsulectomy. Hydrodissection with a dilute epinephrine solution such as tumescent solution is helpful in removing the capsule.

- There is usually very little, if any, capsule over the ADM. I drain this pocket because the radiated tissue will ooze afterward and swelling can last 3 to 4 weeks.
- If the IMF or the lateral fold needs adjustment, I do this with permanent sutures internally and reinforce these with an external through-and-through temporary bolster suture of 1-0-nylon or polypropylene to prevent tearing out the internal sutures.

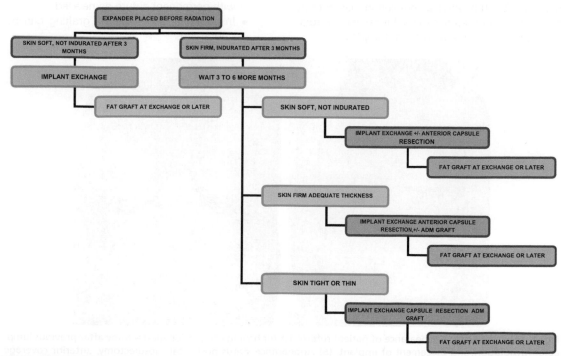

Fig. 2. Algorithm for adjunct procedures done with the implant exchange when the expander is placed before radiation. A similar algorithm is used if the radiation preceded placement of the tissue expander.

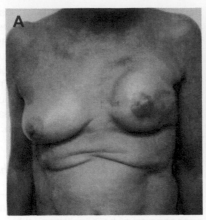
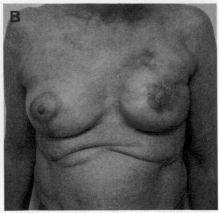

Fig. 3. (*A*) Preoperative appearance of irradiated implant. (*B*) Postoperative appearance after 2-stage procedure: first, placement of acellular dermal matrices (ADM) second, 2 sessions of fat grafting.

- Once the implant has been inserted, I remove the bolster suture.
- A support bra is used 24 hours a day, as possible, for 3 to 4 weeks.

Patients are cautioned about the trade-off of more postoperative pain with the addition of lateral fold sutures into the serratus.

Complex Implant Exchange Procedure

If the skin quality is thick or tight after 9 months postradiation (or 3–6 months after placing an expander in a patient with a previous history of radiation, such as after a completion mastectomy for a recurrence after segmental resection/radiation), the second stage is more complex.

- A complete capsulectomy, rather than an anterior resection only, may be required if the posterior capsule is thick.
- In addition, a second piece of ADM can be added to form a new complete anterior surface or partial anterior surface. If partial, this is usually placed medial and superior.
- External, temporary, marionette sutures are used to guide the ADM into the correct position and then internal tacking sutures of 3-0 absorbable material are used to completely seat the material.
- Pocket border adjustments are sutured with permanent suture as needed.
- In addition, first-stage fat grafting can be performed.

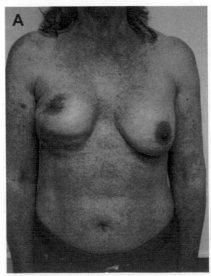
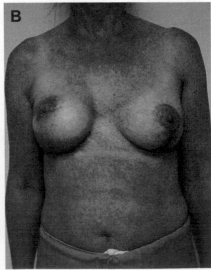

Fig. 4. (*A*) Preoperative appearance of patient referred after having completion mastectomy after previous lumpectomy/radiation and placement of implant. (*B*) Appearance status post total capsulectomy, anterior coverage with ADM, adjustment of IMF, implant replacement, 2 sessions of fat grafting, and left mastopexy. Note the improvement but also the persistence of retracted nipple areola.

Patients are advised that often 2 or 3 sessions of fat grafting done 3 months apart may be needed (**Fig. 3**).

This same concept of capsulectomy, additional ADM, and fat grafting is used in secondary reconstructions of radiated implants in cases where the implant has been already placed (**Fig. 4**). If the capsule is thin or if there is significant rippling, I do not remove it but instead release it as needed and then reinforce with additional ADM and fat graft if needed.

SUMMARY

Radiation to the breast continues to present a difficult problem to the reconstructing plastic surgeon. The effects of radiation on skin and soft tissue can be classified as acute and long term, but there is always permanent impairment to the tissue to some extent. Wound healing in radiated tissue is slower and more prone to dehiscence and/or infection. Prosthetic breast reconstruction that has been irradiated can be compromised aesthetically compared with nonirradiated reconstructions. The addition of ADM to prosthetic breast reconstructions has improved the results and reduced complications compared with those reconstructions without this material that have been irradiated. The author's technique for using ADM is presented in detail. An algorithm is also presented, which assists in thinking about and planning the reconstruction.

REFERENCES

1. Bernstein E, Sullivan F, Mitchell J, et al. Biology of chronic radiation effect on tissues and wound healing. Clin Plast Surg 1993;20(3):435–53.
2. DeMoulin P. A short history of breast cancer. Boston: Martinus Nijhoff; 1983.
3. Lehman M, Hickey B. The less than whole breast radiotherapy approach. Breast 2010;19(3):180–7.
4. Burns J, Mancoll J, Phillips L. Impairments to wound healing. Clin Plast Surg 2003;30(1):47–56.
5. Goodman C, Miller R, Patrick C Jr, et al. Radiotherapy effects on expanded skin. Plast Reconstr Surg 2002;110(4):1080–3.
6. Dvali L, Dagum A, Pang C, et al. Effect of radiation on skin expansion and skin flap viability in pigs. Plast Reconstr Surg 2000;106(3):624–9.
7. Krueger E, Wilkins E, Strawderman M, et al. Complications and patient satisfaction following expander/implant breast reconstruction with and without radiotherapy. Int J Radiat Oncol Biol Phys 2001;49(3):713–21.
8. Christante D, Pommier SE, Diggs B, et al. Using complications associated with postmastectomy radiation and immediate breast reconstruction to

improve surgical decision making. Arch Surg 2010; 145(9):873–8.
9. Vandeweyer E, Deraemaecker R. Radiation therapy after immediate breast reconstruction with implants. Plast Reconstr Surg 2000;106(1):56–8.
10. McCarthy C, Pusic A, Disa J, et al. Unilateral postoperative chest wall radiotherapy in bilateral tissue expander/implant reconstruction patients: a prospective outcomes analysis. Plast Reconstr Surg 2005; 116(6):1642–7.
11. Ascherman J, Hanasono M, Newman M, et al. Implant reconstruction in breast cancer patients treated with radiation therapy. Plast Reconstr Surg 2006;117(2):359–65.
12. Spear S, Onyewu C. Staged breast reconstruction with saline filled implants in the irradiated breast: recent trends and therapeutic implications. Plast Reconstr Surg 2000;105(3):930–42.
13. Parsa A, Jackowe D, Johnson W, et al. Selection criteria for expander/implant breast reconstruction following radiation therapy. Hawaii Med J 2009;68:66–8.
14. Kronowitz S, Hunt K, Kuerer H, et al. Delayed-immediate breast reconstruction. Plast Reconstr Surg 2004;113(6):1617–28.
15. Fine N, Hirsch E. Keeping options open for patients with anticipated postmastectomy chest wall irradiation: immediate tissue expansion followed by reconstruction of choice. Plast Reconstr Surg 2009;123(1):25–9.
16. Cordeiro P, Pusic A, Disa J, et al. Irradiation after immediate tissue expander/implant breast reconstruction: outcomes, complications, aesthetic results, and satisfaction among 156 patients. Plast Reconstr Surg 2004;113(3):877–81.
17. Salzberg C, Ashikari A, Koch R, et al. An 8-year experience of direct to implant immediate breast reconstruction using human acellular dermal matrix (AlloDerm). Plast Reconstr Surg 2011; 127(2):514–24.
18. Breuning K, Warren S. Immediate bilateral breast reconstruction with implants and inferolateral AlloDerm slings. Ann Plast Surg 2005;55(3):232–9.
19. Salzberg A. Nonexpansive immediate breast reconstruction using human acellular tissue matrix graft (AlloDerm). Ann Plast Surg 2006;57(1):1–5.
20. Zienowicz R, Karacaoglu E. Implant-based breast reconstruction with allograft. Plast Reconstr Surg 2007;120(2):373–81.
21. Topol B, Dalton E, Ponn T, et al. Immediate single-stage breast reconstruction using implants and human acellular dermal tissue matrix with adjustment of the lower pole of the breast to reduce unwanted lift. Ann Plast Surg 2008;61(5):494–9.
22. Spear S, Parikh P, Reisin E, et al. Acellular dermis-assisted breast reconstruction. Aesthetic Plast Surg 2008;32:418–25.
23. Losken A. Early results using sterilized acellular human dermis (Neoform) in postmastectomy tissue

expander breast reconstruction. Plast Reconstr Surg 2009;123(6):1654–8.

24. Basu C, Leong M, Hicks M. Acellular cadaveric dermis decreases the inflammatory response in capsule formation in reconstructive breast surgery. Plast Reconstr Surg 2010;126(6):1842–7.

25. Komorowska-Timek E, Oberg K, Timek T, et al. The effect of AlloDerm envelopes on periprosthetic capsule formation with and without radiation. Plast Reconstr Surg 2009;123(3):807–16.

26. Uzunismail A, Duman A, Perk C, et al. The effects of acellular dermal allograft (AlloDerm) interface on silicone-related capsule formation—experimental study. Eur J Plast Surg 2008;31:179–85.

27. Siggelkow W, Faridi A, Spiritus K, et al. Histologic analysis of silicone breast implant capsules and correlation with capsular contracture. Biomaterials 2003;24:1101–9.

28. Newman M, Swartz K, Samson M, et al. The true incidence of near-term postoperative complications in prosthetic breast reconstruction utilizing human acellular dermal matrices: a meta-analysis. Aesthetic Plast Surg 2011;35:100–6.

29. Nahebedian M. AlloDerm performance in the setting of prosthetic breast surgery, infection and irradiation. Plast Reconstr Surg 2009;124(6):1743–53.

30. Seruya M, Cohen M, Rao S, et al. Two-stage prosthetic breast reconstruction using AlloDerm: a 7-year experience in irradiated and nonirradiated breasts [abstract]. Plast Reconstr Surg 2010;126(Suppl 4):22–3.

31. Coleman S. Structural fat grafting. St Louis (MO): Quality Medical Publishing; 2004.

32. Rigotti G, Marchi A, Galie' M, et al. Clinical treatment of radiotherapy tissue damage by lipoaspirate transplant: a healing process mediated by adipose-derived adult stem cells. Plast Reconstr Surg 2007;119(5):1409–22.

33. Serra-Renom J, Munoz-Olmo J, Serra-Mestre J. Fat grafting in postmastectomy breast reconstruction with expanders and prostheses in patients who have received radiotherapy: formation of new subcutaneous tissue. Plast Reconstr Surg 2010;125(1):12–8.

Emerging Applications for Acellular Dermal Matrices in Mastopexy

Bradley P. Bengtson, MD[a],*, Richard A. Baxter, MD[b,c]

KEYWORDS

- Acellular dermal matrix • Mastopexy
- Periareolar mastopexy • Strattice™ • AlloDerm®
- Mesh mastopexy • ADM • Revision augmentation

Key Points

- Meshed acellular dermal matrix (ADM) as an internal bra may help prevent bottoming out and maintain upper pole fullness over the long term after mastopexy.
- Early experience shows a potentially useful application of ADM donut- or washer-shaped grafts in revision periareolar mastopexy.
- ADM grafts for periareolar mastopexy may prevent areolar widening and unfavorable scarring.
- Permanent suture and mesh materials for mastopexy support may be complicated by biofilms, infections, and other late-presenting problems not associated with ADMs.

Acellular dermal matrices (ADMs), originally developed for the treatment of burn patients, are now an important emerging technology in complex hernia repair, orthopedics, breast reconstruction and now revision aesthetic surgery of the breast. Their use in breast reconstruction and cosmetic breast revision was, in retrospect a fortuitous development. Although Level 1 evidence is lacking and is increasing, ADMs have unquestionably become helpful adjuncts for these applications. As techniques and best practices have developed, the array of uses expanded from revision surgery to primary implant-based reconstruction, and from simple capsule reinforcement to repair of fold malpositions and animation deformity. New applications continue to be explored, some of which are described in this article. However, these are in early stages of development and their long-term value remains to be demonstrated.

GENERAL CONSIDERATIONS IN MASTOPEXY

Although a popular procedure, mastopexy continues to be plagued by long-term loss of upper pole fullness

Disclosures: Dr Bengtson is a consultant for Allergan Medical and LifeCell Corporation/KCI; a lead investigator for Natrelle Style 410 cohesive gel implant studies: Core and Continued Access; an investigator for Allergan responsive gel and Mentor gel core and adjunct studies; and an Aesthetic Surgery Education and Research Foundation (ASERF) grant recipient for high resolution ultrasound research.
Dr Baxter is a consultant and speaker for LifeCell Corporation and Allergan Breast Aesthetics, and an investigator for Sientra, Inc.
[a] Bengtson Center for Aesthetics and Plastic Surgery, 555 MidTowne Street NE, Suite 110, Grand Rapids, MI 49503, USA
[b] Private Practice, Seattle, WA, USA
[c] Plastic Surgery Clinic, 6100 219th Street SW, Suite 290, Mountlake Terrace, WA 98043, USA
* Corresponding author.
E-mail address: drb@bengtsoncenter.com

Clin Plastic Surg 39 (2012) 159–166
doi:10.1016/j.cps.2012.02.006
0094-1298/12/$ – see front matter © 2012 Elsevier Inc. All rights reserved.

despite early good results.[1] Mastopexy was initially conceived as a skin reshaping operation, with parenchyma adapting passively to the skin envelope.[2,3] Results with these techniques were generally satisfactory and they became the standard approach for several years. Mastopexy techniques are still described according to the cutaneous scar configuration.[4] However, the push to short scar techniques prompted a focus on parenchymal reshaping and less reliance on the skin envelope for support.[5] Nevertheless, these may also relapse over time, and more extensive parenchymal dissection and mobilization in an attempt to enhance projection and upper pole fullness is not always an optimal solution.

An internal bra composed of deepithelialized dermis has been proposed as a means of maintaining shape while limiting tension on the skin envelope. However, because of the surface area required, it is suitable primarily for cases of "remarkable hypertrophy or severe ptosis"[6] and has not become popular. Dermal bra procedures are generally limited to Wise pattern mastopexy, and are less appropriate for limited scar techniques.

Because of these difficulties in maintaining shape and projection, various mesh materials have been tried for additional support. Polypropylene mesh was used as early as 1981 with reduction mammaplasty.[7] With the introduction of short scar techniques, the concept of an internal mesh bra in the subcutaneous layer was developed. Absorbable mesh has been used, with the hope that a scar layer would form in the configuration of the mesh bra, but this technique did not produce long-lasting results with periareolar mastopexy.[8] In an attempt to maintain shape, a mixed mesh (40% polyester, 60% absorbable polyglactin) was used with reportedly better results, although long-term follow-up was not specified.[9] Preshaped polyester mesh has also been used with reported success.[10] Follow-up histology showed a mechanically strong but supple mesh with collagen ingrowth.[11] Despite the success reported by some,

other reports have shown that a permanent foreign body in the subcutaneous layer of the breast may be subject to biofilm and infection.[12] These types of concerns about synthetic mesh in the breast have limited its adoption.

The use of autologous or cadaveric dermal slings for mastopexy mesh was reported by Colwell and Breuing[13] in a series of 10 patients, 5 in each category. The authors proposed an algorithm for selecting either autologous tissue or ADM based on the quantity and quality of skin available. Results were stable at 6 months to 3 years in this series, indicating that tissue-based mesh could provide an alternative to synthetic mesh and durable results (**Fig. 1**).

An acellular product, FortaPerm (Organogenesis, Canton, MA, USA), has also been used with periareolar mastopexy.[14] FortaPerm is a highly crosslinked and laminated material derived from porcine intestinal submucosa, and its primary application is in urology, where it has been used for pubovaginal slings.[15] It is believed to be slowly resorbed and replaced with a native collagen layer. For mastopexy support, the material is passed through a Zimmer mesher and the entire breast is wrapped. The ideal product would be noninflammatory and biocompatible, such as ADM, so it can be incorporated without loss of integrity.

PATIENT SELECTION FOR ADM FOR MASTOPEXY

Given the high cost of ADM materials, their use will likely become routine for primary mastopexy, despite the variability of long-term stability of shape and projection with standard techniques. However, for cases of recurrent ptosis or pseudoptosis, the use of a mesh bra provides an option. In the case of augmentation mastopexy with bottoming out, the use of ADM is well-established, so its use for mastopexy without implants represents an extension of the same

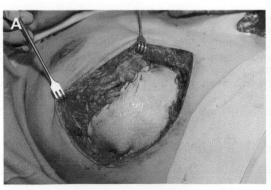
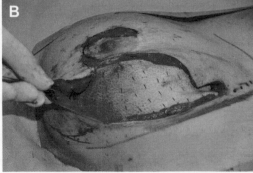

Fig. 1. (*A, B*) Dermal slings for mastopexy mesh.

concept. Patients who have experienced massive weight loss may have atrophic tissues despite an abundance of extra skin available for use as an autologous graft. In this sense, the same principle applies to patients receiving an implant and those with ptosis: replacing "like with like" through using a connective tissue matrix to reinforce weakened tissues that provide inadequate support. In addition, the cellular tissue requirements of an autogenous tissue are more demanding than those of the acellular dermal–collagen construct that ADMs provide, and also obviate the problems associated with thin, nonuniform pieces when trying to use the patient's own tissues.

TECHNICAL POINTS: MASTOPEXY HAMMOCK

Given the limited experience with ADM mesh for mastopexy support, technical considerations are still evolving. A primary concern is selection of the appropriate ADM material. In expander/implant reconstruction, human-derived ADM may be favored because of its potential to expand, but this may be a counterproductive property for ptosis repair. For that reason, porcine-derived materials such as Strattice™ (LifeCell Corporation, Branchburg, NJ, USA) may be preferable. These materials are relatively inelastic and used for abdominal wall repair and revision implant surgery. However, the ability of porcine-derived ADM to conform to a three-dimensional contour is limited for the same reason. A premeshed version may become available, but a series of incisions with a #15 blade can suffice to expand and modify the product to some degree (**Fig. 2**). Perforating may also improve the "take" of the material or minimize the risk of seroma formation in the subcutaneous plane, but too much may weaken it.

A critical decision in planning is the size and shape of the ADM. For a periareolar mastopexy, totally encasing the parenchymal mound in a cone of ADM may be required for optimal projection, as is done with synthetic and composite mesh materials using the Góes method. Most cases will probably only require a sling across the lower pole, analogous to a demi cup bra. Further experience will help refine the process for selecting the optimal size and orientation.

To provide fixation of the mesh at the boundaries of the breast mound, adequate undermining is required. Vigilance in attention to flap thickness is necessary because of the wider undermining. Fixation to chest wall is necessary unless the mesh is used only for shaping, but generally, setting the inframammary, medial, and lateral folds is helpful and necessary if a sling effect is desired. If possible, a cuff of the graft a few millimeters wide is splayed onto the chest wall and sutured with #00 polydioxanone or similar resorbable material. The anterior or superior edge may be sutured directly to the parenchyma or deepithelialized dermis. Sitting the patient upright to asses shape is critical before final tailoring and adjustments. Matching the internal bra to the skin envelope in the upright position avoids irregularities from redundancy and overresection leading to tension on the closure.

Periareolar Mastopexy

Periareolar mastopexy has a long history in breast surgery, dating back to the 1970s according to recent literature.[16–18] Since its inception, it has been associated with a wide variety of complications or at least issues that have made it less than ideal with surgeons mainly adding a vertical component or looking at other techniques. These issues were well reviewed by Spear and colleagues in 1990[19] and 2001.[20] As described, Góes has used the periareolar approach but also adds gland reshaping, and often uses internal mesh support to help hold the gland in position and remove periareolar tension. Hammond and colleagues[21] described an excellent and intriguing

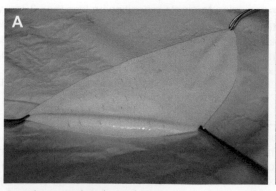
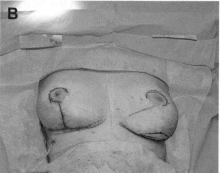

Fig. 2. Strattice™ porcine-derived ADM with multiple perforations from a #15 blade for use in mastopexy support.

technique of an interlocking polytetrafluoroethylene (Gore-Tex; W. L. Gore & Associates, Inc., Flagstaff, AZ, USA) suture that can maintain nice areolar shape but still has the potential for Biofilm, extrusion, and suture track infection. Secondary to these limitations, many surgeons, except in minimal nipple repositioning, have added a vertical component that helps limit the flattening from a periareolar mastopexy alone, unless some additional breast shaping is performed.

ADMs

Beginning with AlloDerm® in treating complex burn wounds and now extending into multiple uses and subspecialties, a multitude of ADMs are now being used in reconstructive breast surgery and a wide variety of ever-increasing applications across surgical specialties. As described throughout this issue of *Clinics in Plastic Surgery,* ADMs are being used to correct a wide variety of aesthetic breast complications, including malposition, stretch deformity, coverage issues of wrinkling and rippling, and capsular contracture among others. In only a matter of time they will make their way into primary breast procedures, and they have already been implemented primarily for breast reductions/mastopexies as an internal sling or hammock. This section reviews early experience with the use of a periareolar piece alone to provide support and long-term maintenance of areolar diameter.

METHODS

For the use of donut-shaped grafts in periareolar mastopexy, cadaver laboratory studies were performed to determine the feasibility, best range of sizes, technical factors, and break strength. These studies were followed by a small clinical feasibility study with a 1 year maximum follow-up. A 3-cm inner circle diameter and 5.5-cm outer diameter of Strattice™ was inset as a "washer" after deepithelialization was performed. The outer diameter dermis was then sutured through the Strattice™/AlloDerm® at either 38 to 40 mm from the center of the nipple and then through the inner areolar dermis. Average nipple elevation was 2.5 cm, and four revision and four primary mastopexy breasts were performed.

In Vitro Studies

The authors first began in the cadaver laboratory testing various shapes, sizes, and materials. The inner diameter is deceptively large in position and the authors believed that a size of approximately 3 cm allowed for the material to be placed

under the areola without extensive undermining. The outer diameter size range the authors judged to be ideal was closest to 5.5 cm (**Fig. 3**A). This diameter allows for lateral stability without the material buckling or folding back on itself, and extensive undermining is unnecessary (see **Fig. 3**B).

- The ADM was secured internally at the 3, 6, 9, and 12 o'clock positions with a 3-0 - poliglecaprone suture (Monocryl; Ethicon, Inc., Somerville, NJ, USA), at the periphery at the same points, and one additional suture between each quadrant.
- The ADM is then marked at 40 mm from the center or 1 cm outside the inner margin.
- The closure is then begun by grabbing the dermis of the outer diameter, placing a superficial skiving bite through the ADM at the 38 to 40 mm marked point, and then suturing the inner dermal areolar margin again at 3, 6, 9, 12 o'clock with a 3-0 Monocryl and at halfway points (see **Fig. 3**C).
- Next a 3-0 polyglycolide-poly-e-caprolactone copolymer suture (Monoderm Quill, Angiotech, Reading, PA, USA) is run, with the same sequence completing the closure. The quill is nice in that it can help create a slightly irregular border, mimicking more of an irregular areolar margin (see **Fig. 3**D).

The tension and bursting strength required in the laboratory, although not measured with any specific devices, is nearly impossible to break with excessive lateral pull after the closure is completed.

Satisfied with the basic technique refinements, the authors offered this repair to a small series of patients as an off-label application of the product. The company offered the product complimentary to the patient.

A series of eight patients elected this approach over the past year. The authors limited the inclusion to nipple repositioning less than 3 cm, which is their current criteria for offering this technique before transitioning to a circumvertical pattern. The average nipple elevation was 2.5 cm, and three patients had primary mastopexy and three were revision, with one in each group a bilateral mastopexy.

Early Clinical Results

Results have been good, with an average range of stretch from 0 to 8 mm postoperatively, with up to 1 year follow-up, 7-month average (**Table 1**). One patient had a suture track infection, necessitating

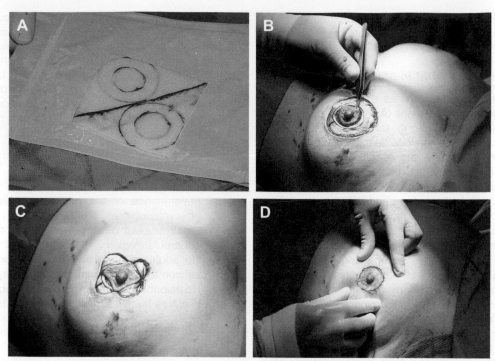

Fig. 3. (*A*) An 8 × 8 cm Strattice™ ADM graft marked for two donut pieces. (*B*) Placement of graft. (*C*) Closure at 3, 6, 9, and 12 o'clock positions before pursestring suture. (*D*) After closure with barbed suture.

removal of the nonintegrated ADM. This occurrence encouraged the authors to place a large Op-Site over the breast, leaving the nipple exposed to apply some external pressure and support the ADM through healing and minimizing activity with a sports bra for 4 weeks. Good ADM incorporation and no major infections, other exposures, extrusions, or significant hypertrophic scarring were seen with up to a 1-year follow-up.

The cadaver laboratory showed that the inner diameter required is somewhat smaller than anticipated, with the optimal range being approximately 3 cm and the outer diameter approximately 5.5 cm diameter. The goals are to provide enough of a base beneath the areolar margin but not devascularize the nipple, and to provide enough lateral support but not have the ADM fold back on itself. The restretch postoperatively was minimal in the first eight patients, with the average areolar diameter postoperatively being 44 mm (range, 38–48), with an average follow-up of 7 months, and restretch being 0 to 8 mm

Table 1
Areolar measurements with ADM donut/washer technique[a]

Breast # Period	Areolar Diameter Preoperatively	NAR set@ Surgery	NAR Postoperatively	Postoperative
1	58 mm × 56 mm	40 mm	43 mm	12 mo
2	65 mm × 60 mm	40 mm	44 mm	10 mo
3	62 mm × 60 mm	40 mm	48 mm	8 mo
4	68 mm × 60 mm	40 mm	42 mm	8 mo
5	48 mm × 55 mm	38 mm	38 mm	6 mo
6	48 mm × 50 mm	38 mm	46 mm	5 mo
7	75 mm × 70 mm	40 mm	44 mm	4 mo
8	56 mm × 60 mm	40 mm	42 mm	3 mo

Abbreviation: NAR, nipple areolar reconstruction.
[a] Primary author early series.

(**Fig. 4** for preoperative and postoperative patient views). An average of 15 minutes was added to the mean operating time.

Discussion of ADM in Mastopexy

Periareolar mastopexy as a stand-alone procedure continues to be one of the least popular mastopexy options among many plastic surgeons because of the limitations described with recurrent stretch, breast flattening, palpability, or suture track infection necessitating removal. Moreover, areolar diameter is not static but rather affected by factors such as temperature and stimulation. Fixation with a synthetic material interferes with this, so that instead of radial expansion and contraction, the nipple–areolar complex may seem to herniated ("Snoopy dog" deformity). A biologic material that becomes integrated may be more likely to perform as normal tissues while still preventing long-term expansion. Avoidance of a nondistensible purse-string suture will also prevent palpability, but use of resorbable materials leads to reexpansion to variable degrees.

ADMs are moving from purely reconstructive procedures into cosmetic applications in both revision and now occasionally primary aesthetic operations. Use of ADMs is quickly becoming standard for recurrent breast revision complications, such as malposition, stretch deformities,

wrinkling, and rippling, and for reducing recurrent capsular contraction. They have also be used in augmentation mastopexy and reductions for patients who have sustained massive weight loss as internal hammocks and slings to support breast tissue and relieve the load and pressure on the lower breast. Whoever controls the lower pole of the breast maintaining the distance from nipple to inframammary fold controls the breast result over time.

Potential benefits of this periareolar ADM-assisted mastopexy include:

- Maintenance of the periareolar diameter after mastopexy
- Small amount of added projection to the subareolar region
- No additional vertical component or conversion to a circumvertical mastopexy
- No palpable periareolar suture with decrease in suture track infection.

Disadvantages of this technique include:

- Additional cost of the product
- Slight increase in surgical time
- Potential for extrusion or infection until revascularization.

Potential exists for using extra tissue obtained in processing of the ADM, which may decrease

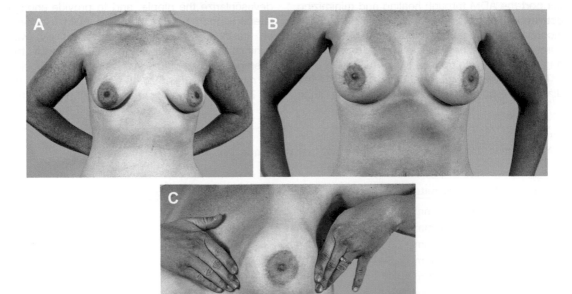

Fig. 4. (*A*) Preoperative view. (*B*) 1-Year postoperatively. (*C*) Close-up of postoperative view.

standard cost structure, and if extra tissue is available when using a larger piece for another part of the procedure and a patient requires a minimal mastopexy, this technique should be considered. In contrast to only revascularizing from one surface in most breast revisions and reconstructions, this technique has the advantage of revascularizing from both the superficial and deep surfaces so that delays or wound healing problems may be minimized.

The new reverse cutting needles are very sharp and do not dull during the repair. If increased stretch does occur over time, consideration for a longer lasting or permanent suture such as 3-0 or 4-0 Ethibond, at the 3, 6, 9, and 12 o'clock and intervening positions. Additional ADMs placed over a mastopexy buttress or pillar repair could also be considered.

CONCLUSIONS

With limited experience to date, the application of ADM materials in mastopexy is still emerging, but holds promise. For revision procedures, the rationale for its use is supported by considerable experience in related breast implant–based procedures, which may extrapolate to mastopexy without implants because the need for lower pole support is the same. Currently, indications for their use are not rigidly defined and require judgment, and further studies are needed. The donut graft for periareolar mastopexy seems to be a useful procedure for both primary and revision procedures based on preliminary data.

SUMMARY

Meshed ADM grafts seem useful in supporting mastopexies to minimize the chances of bottoming out and loss of upper pole projection. For periareolar mastopexy, the authors believe they have a good dimensional size for the "washer" piece of the ADM. The actual set diameter may be altered by the surgeon and at patient request, but it is typically set at 38 to 40 mm. This method adds potential projection to the areola; holds with acceptable range of restretch, certainly much better than conventional simple periareolar nonweave mastopexies; and adds minimal time to the procedure (an average of 15 minutes). Although very early in the healing process, it may provide another option in maintaining nipple–areolar diameter long-term. The authors had one patient with a suture track infection necessitating removal of the unincorporated material, and some adjustments in the intraoperative and postoperative course were subsequently made and continue to evolve.

REFERENCES

1. Spear SL, Low M, Ducic I. Revision augmentation mastopexy: indications, operations, and outcomes. Ann Plast Surg 2003;51(6):540–6.
2. Goulian D. Dermal mastopexy. Plast Reconstr Surg 1971;47(2):105–10.
3. Strombeck JO. Mammaplasty: report of a new technique based on the two pedicle principle. Br J Plast Surg 1960;13:79.
4. Rohrich RJ, Gosman AA, Brown SA, et al. Mastopexy preferences: a survey of board-certified plastic surgeons. Plast Reconstr Surg 2006;118(7):1631–8.
5. Hall-Findlay EJ. Pedicles in vertical breast reduction and mastopexy. Clin Plast Surg 2002;29(3):379–91.
6. Qiao Q, Sun J, Liu C, et al. Reduction mammaplasty and correction of ptosis: dermal bra technique. Plast Reconstr Surg 2003;111(3):1122–30.
7. Johnson GW. Central core reduction mammaplasties and Marlex suspension of breast tissue. Aesthetic Plast Surg 1981;5(1):77–84.
8. Góes JC. Periareolar mammaplasty: double skin technique with application of polyglactine 910 mesh. Rev Soc Bras Cir Plas 1992;7:1–3.
9. Góes JC. Periareolar mastopexy: double skin technique with mesh support. Aesthetic Surg J 2003;23(2):129–35.
10. deBruijn HP, Johannes S. Mastopexy with 3D preshaped mesh for long-term results: development of the internal bra system. Aesthetic Plast Surg 2008;32:757–65.
11. deBruijn HP, ten Thije RH, Johannes S. Mastopexy with mesh reinforcement: the mechanical characteristics of polyester mesh in the female breast. Plast Reconstr Surg 2009;124(2):364–71.
12. Dixon JM, Arnott I, Schaverian M. Chronic abscess formation following mesh mastopexy: case report. J Plast Reconstr Aesthet Surg 2010;63(7):1220–2.
13. Colwell AS, Breuing KH. Improving shape and symmetry in mastopexy with autologous or cadaveric dermal slings. Ann Plast Surg 2008;61(2):138–42.
14. Góes JC, Bates D. Periareolar mastopexy with Forta-Perm. Aesthetic Plast Surg 2010;34(3):350–8.
15. Santucci RA, Barber TD. Resorbable extracellular matrix grafts in urologic reconstruction. Int Braz J Urol 2005;31(3):192–203.
16. Andrews JM, Aoki-Yshizuki MM, Martins DM, et al. An areolar approach to reduction mammaplasty. Br J Plast Surg 1975;28(3):166–70.
17. Bartels RJ, Strickland DM, Douglas WM. A new mastopexy operation for mild or moderate breast ptosis. Plast Reconstr Surg 1976;57(6):687–91.

18. Gruber RP, Jones HW Jr. The "donut" mastopexy: indications and complications. Plast Reconstr Surg 1980;65(1):34–8.

19. Spear SL, Kassan M, Little JW. Guidelines in concentric mastopexy. Plast Reconstr Surg 1990;85(6):961–6.

20. Spear SL, Giese SY, Ducic I. Concentric mastopexy revisited. Plast Reconstr Surg 2001;107(5):1294–9.

21. Hammond DC, Khuthaila DK, Kim J. The interlocking Gore-tex suture for control of areolar diameter and shape. Plast Reconstr Surg 2007;119(3):804–9.

Comparison of Different ADM Materials in Breast Surgery

Angela Cheng, MD, Michel Saint-Cyr, MD, FRCS*

KEYWORDS

- ADM/acellular dermal matrix • AlloDerm® • Strattice™
- DermACELL™ • FlexHD® • DermaMatrix®
- AlloMax™ • SurgiMend®

Key Points

- Alloderm is the most well supported ADM, with abundant evidence and historical experience among plastic reconstructive surgeons.
- Surgeons should be aware if a selected ADM requires orientation and be able to distinguish the different sides.
- Human-based products likely result in a less inflammatory reaction.
- Several ADMs are actually aseptic and NOT sterile, which may be a factor contributing to the increased risk of infection with ADM use in expander-based reconstruction.
- AlloDerm® and DermACELL™ are exposed to antibiotics during processing and, therefore, patient allergies and sensitivities should be considered before implantation.
- Newer ADMs require less rehydration/rinsing in preparation for use.
- The use of ADMs in breast reconstruction is gaining popularity but may not be covered by insurance. Submitting for preapproval is critical to avoid significant costs to patients.

ADM OPTIONS

Breast reconstruction continues to evolve and, for many surgeons, now frequently incorporates use of a variety of acellular dermal matrices (ADMs), especially for lower-lateral coverage of implants, nipple reconstruction, secondary correction of breast deformities, and reinforcement of the abdominal donor defects in autologous tissue reconstruction. The introduction of these ADMs has facilitated immediate implant reconstruction. Advantages versus complete submuscular coverage include improved implant positioning via defining the inframammary and lateral mammary fold, preventing window-shading of the pectoralis muscle, serving as an internal support, shorter expansion times, and even protective effects against radiation changes.[1–4] ADMs have also advanced correction of secondary breast deformities, including minimizing bottoming out, masking implant rippling, treating capsular contracture, addressing malposition, and compensating for overlying soft tissue deficiency.[5] Concerns about using ADMs have included potential increases in infection, inflammatory reaction, seroma, masking

---

Disclosure: Dr Michel Saint-Cyr is a consultant for LifeCell, Mentor, and Allergan.
Department of Plastic Surgery, UT Southwestern Medical Center, 1801 Inwood Road, Dallas, TX 75390-9132, USA
* Corresponding author.
E-mail address: MSaintCyr@me.com

Clin Plastic Surg 39 (2012) 167–175
doi:10.1016/j.cps.2012.02.004
0094-1298/12/$ – see front matter Published by Elsevier Inc.

or mimicking tumor recurrence, and obviously cost.[6–9]

The diversity of available tissue products poses a significant challenge to reconstructive breast surgeons trying to select an optimal ADM and few data exist to compare these products directly. Many of the earliest studies were performed using animal models by each manufacturer and not only are the data unpublished but also they may not correlate with in vivo performance. The existing published data are mostly based on reconstruction of abdominal wall or hernia repair, which cannot necessarily be extrapolated to breast reconstruction. These products vary in many aspects, including the source of tissue, processing, storage, surgical preparation, available sizes, and cost. Several ADMs claim added benefit of cross-linking, a process that may improve the long-term tensile strength but also potentially results in an increase in foreign body reaction and encapsulation. A final consideration involves the limitations of individual insurance coverage, which may vary for each of these products. Although AlloDerm® is gaining acceptance, many of these other ADMs are considered experimental and may result in substantial costs passed onto patients, which should be taken into consideration when submitting for insurance preapproval.

ALLODERM® (LIFECELL)

Probably the most familiar product to most plastic surgeons, AlloDerm® was the first human dermis product available in 1994. Despite the initial indication for burn coverage, it has been subsequently expanded into a variety of applications, including abdominal wall reconstruction, head and neck reconstruction, and breast reconstruction. Early success has translated into widespread popularity among plastic and reconstructive surgeons, with the first reported case of its use in breast reconstruction in 2005 as an inferolateral sling.[10] This was followed shortly thereafter with a report on the use of acellular cadaveric dermis with expander-based reconstruction.[11] Today, Allo-Derm has even been used as an adjunct for nipple reconstruction.[12,13]

AlloDerm® Storage and Preparation

AlloDerm® Regenerative Tissue Matrix is a cadaveric split-thickness skin graft that is aseptically processed with sodium chloride and sodium deoxycholate and freeze-dried. It is supplied in an inner (Tyvek) pouch, which is not sterile. The package labeling, originally indicating refrigeration at 1°C to 25°C (34°F–77°F), was required to ensure the labeled shelf life, a significant distinguishing factor

from other products. In a recent statement released by the manufacturer on July 14, 2010, however, the manufacturer found no deleterious effects on graft performance in animal models after exposure of −30°C (−22°F) for 10 days and 60°C (140°F) for 45 days. The product should not be used if bent, broken, or cracked before rehydration, which may require 10 to 40 minutes, another clinically noteworthy inconvenience. The AlloDerm® itself should not be further sterilized. The manufacturer recommends submerging the tissue completely for a minimum of 5 minutes or until the backing separates in warm (up to 37°C) normal saline or lactated Ringer solution with gentle agitation, then transferring to a second bath, which can include antibiotics until fully rehydrated and pliable. The matrix must then be used within 4 hours of rehydration.

The newest available product is AlloDerm® Regenerative Tissue Matrix (RTM) *Ready to use* which does not require refrigeration or rehydration. The inner pouch is actually sterile and the product is terminally sterilized to a Sterility Assurance Level of 10^{-3}.

AlloDerm® Use in Surgical Implantation

AlloDerm® has 2 distinct surfaces and, therefore, requires attention to orientation during surgical implantation. The dermal side of the product is easily recognized by the dull, rough texture and bloodstained appearance when in contact with blood. This is generally placed against the more vascularized wound bed or tissue, such as mastectomy skin flaps, to improve revascularization. Premeshed grafts actually contain a letter "L" in the mesh pattern, which is visible in the proper orientation when the basement membrane side is up.[14] When used for implant-based reconstruction, the manufacturer recommends 2 drains, one between the implant and AlloDerm® and another underneath the skin flap, but commonly only a single drain is placed above the AlloDerm® and beneath the mastectomy flap.[15] The matrix is available in a variety of sizes and thicknesses ranging from 0.23 mm to 3.30 mm. Large sheets are available in a range from 4 cm × 12 cm to 16 cm × 20 cm for the implantable thick and X-thick products (1.04–2.28 mm and 2.30–3.30 mm, respectively).

Contraindications for AlloDerm® Use

An under-recognized issue with AlloDerm® pertains to the contraindications. During the processing of tissue, a variety of antibiotics are used and, theoretically, exclude any patient sensitive to any of the antibiotics listed on the package or to Polysorbate 20, used in the buffer solution.

AlloDerm® Literature Reviews

AlloDerm® has also been studied extensively, with 515 references in the PubMed database, including 57 related to breast reconstruction. The technique of breast reconstruction using AlloDerm® is well described by Spear and colleagues in *Surgery of the Breast: Principles and Art.*[16] LifeCell has spent 4 years developing a novel primate model 92% homologous to humans to further evaluate the immune response of ADMs beyond the 4 weeks after which other animal models form cross-species reactions.[17] AlloDerm® has also been reported to reconstruct the abdominal wall fascial defects after abdominal-based flap reconstruction.[18] Unlike other newer products, AlloDerm® has reported long-term follow-up addressing complications[19] and evidence that it does not interfere with postoperative radiographic evaluation.[20] A recent review series by Jansen and Macadam[21] found 93% of the studies only level IV evidence but an overall lower rate of capsular contracture when compared to cases without Allo-Derm. A subsequent cost analysis justified the use of AlloDerm® for direct-to-implant breast reconstruction.[22] AlloDerm® has served as a pioneer in the application of ADMs for breast reconstruction and newer ADMs lag behind in supportive evidence at this time.

STRATTICE™ (LIFECELL)

A more recently introduced product of LifeCell, Strattice™ Reconstructive Tissue Matrix, is a terminally sterilized, processed porcine dermis. The matrix is preserved in a phosphate-buffered aqueous solution with stabilizers designed to minimize tissue attachment, which is more advantageous in hernia repair to minimize adhesions, but effects on capsule formation are unclear.

Strattice™ Storage and Preparation

This product is stored at room temperature but the surgical preparation requires only 2 minutes of soaking in room temperature saline or lactated Ringer solution because it is fully hydrated in the original packaging and should be discarded if it is dry when opened. Similar to AlloDerm®, the inner package is not sterile and the tissue must be removed with sterile forceps. Strattice™ is supplied in 2 versions (pliable and firm) and only a single thickness, which ranges from 1.5 to 2.0 mm. The smallest available size is 6 cm × 8 cm with the largest available up to 25 cm × 40 cm, which is a huge advantage for large abdominal wall defects. The 6 cm × 8 cm, 5 cm × 16 cm, and 8 cm × 16 cm pliable sheets are recommended for breast reconstruction.

Contraindications for Strattice™ Use

Strattice™ is contraindicated in patients with sensitivities to porcine material or Polysorbate 20.[23]

Strattice™ Literature Reviews

Only 11 citations in PubMed are available regarding Strattice™. In a direct comparison of a human Allo-Derm versus Strattice™ for hernia repair, Campbell and colleagues[24] found less cellular and vascular infiltration in Strattice™ but improved tensile strength at 4 weeks. Although this is beneficial for hernia repair, vascularized tissue is critical to preventing infection whenever a breast prosthesis is placed. A single case report on histologic analysis of Strattice™ in breast reconstruction with an expander describes intraoperative adherence to the pectoralis muscle and overlying soft tissues. Biopsy demonstrated mild fibroblastic reaction with focal tissue integration at 6 weeks but there were areas within the Strattice™ in which angiogenesis could not be demonstrated.[25]

DERMAMATRIX® (SYNTHES/MUSCULOSKELETAL TRANSPLANT FOUNDATION)

DermaMatrix® is an acellular human dermis product processed by the Musculoskeletal Transplant Foundation (MTF) and available through Synthes. The tissue is processed with sodium chloride and detergent to remove the epidermis and viable dermal cells, then disinfected with acidic and antiseptic reagents so that it passes the United States Pharmacopeia Standard 71 for sterility. The final process involves freeze-drying.

DermaMatrix® Storage and Preparation

Because it is freeze-dried, the product must be rehydrated in room temperature saline or lactated Ringer solution, which can take up to 3 minutes. The inner package can be placed directly onto the sterile field. To facilitate proper orientation, a notch is located in the upper left corner when the epidermal or basement membrane side is facing up. There are 4 available thicknesses (0.2–4 mm, 0.4–0.8 mm, 0.8–1.7 mm, and 1.7+ mm), which vary in sizes from 1 cm × 2 cm to 6 cm × 16 cm. DermaMatrix® is not recommended in patients with autoimmune connective tissue disease.[26]

DermaMatrix® Literature Reviews

A review of published studies via a PubMed search for DermaMatrix® yielded only 8 results. In a 2008 study comparing AlloDerm® with DermaMatrix® in immediate expander-based breast reconstruction, 30 patients (50 breasts) were divided into 2 cohorts.

The only statistically significant difference was in the average number of days the drains were in place, 11 for AlloDerm® versus 13 for DermaMatrix®. The investigators reported a shorter time to final expansion, larger incremental volumes of expansion, and larger final expanded volumes with DermaMatrix® but no difference between the final expanded volume-to-implant ratio. No histologic difference in vascularity was appreciated. Anecdotally, the investigators reported AlloDerm® more elastic and pliable. No differences in complication rates, such as wound infection or seroma, were noted.[27] Another study comparing 4 soft tissue substrates implanted in a submuscular murine model found AlloDerm® became spherical and softer whereas DermaMatrix® retained its shape and consistency.[28]

FLEXHD® (ETHICON/MUSCULOSKELETAL TRANSPLANT FOUNDATION)

FlexHD® is another human allograft matrix that is minimally processed to remove the epidermal and dermal cells and available through an alliance with MTF and Ethicon. The tissue is soaked in a hypertonic solution to remove the cellular elements and rinsed with a detergent and then a proprietary disinfectant before packaging in a 70% ethanol solution. There may be trace amounts of residual ethanol on the product but no antibiotic contamination, which minimizes the potential risks of any sensitivities to antibiotic exposure. FlexHD® cannot be subject to additional sterilization procedures.

FlexHD® Storage and Preparation

The product is prehydrated and does not require refrigeration. A sterilized foil pouch is contained within the Tyvek package. If not used immediately within 30 minutes, the product should be maintained in a sterile saline bath and implanted or discarded within 24 hours. Similar to AlloDerm®, the tissue must be oriented and there should be an indicating notch in the upper left side. The product is available in 3 different thicknesses: thin (0.4–0.8 mm), thick (0.8–1.7 mm), and ultrathick (1.8 mm), with variable sizes from 1 cm × 2 cm for implantation to a maximal size of 20 cm × 25 cm. A specific breast package is available for purchase in bilateral reconstruction, which offers a slight financial discount. FlexHD® is not recommended in patients with autoimmune connective tissue disease.[29]

FlexHD® Literature Review

A brief search on PubMed for FlexHD® generated only 3 results. One in vivo study using FlexHD® and AlloDerm® for hernia repair in a rabbit model demonstrated similar tensile strength.[30] In a different in vitro study, FlexHD® induced significantly more interleukin-1β, an inflammatory cytokine produced by activated macrophages, than AlloMax™ and AlloDerm®.[31]

PERMACOL™ (COVIDIEN)

The Permacol™ implant was introduced by Covidien as a sheet of porcine dermal collagen, which has been processed to remove cellular elements and then cross-linked with hexamethylene diisocyanate to improve the tensile strength and therefore long-term durability. The cross-linking process affects the individual collagen strands of triple helix at lysine and hydroxylysine residues, which slows the breakdown of the collagen scaffold by collagenase. The product is less pliable than other matrices and not recommended for breast reconstruction.

Permacol™ Storage and Preparation

Available for use off the shelf, this product requires no rehydration or refrigeration and is terminally sterilized with γ-irradiation. The ease of rapid availability for use is a definite advantage compared with other existing ADMs. The inner pouch is sterile and ready to be placed onto the sterile field. The manufacturer does recommend that the opened implant be placed into a basin of sterile saline to prevent it from drying out because it cannot be rehydrated. The product does not require any special orientation or positioning and is available is a large range of sizes, from 1 cm × 4 cm × 0.5 cm to 28 cm × 40 cm × 1.5 cm. The exceptionally large sheets are a distinct advantage especially for abdominal wall reconstruction but less of a concern for breast surgery. Permacol™ is not recommended for breast reconstruction, because it does not provide adequate laxity to achieve natural, ptotic lower pole coverage. The manufacturer does not list any absolute contraindications.[32]

Permacol™ Literature Reviews

Permacol™ was studied as a soft tissue implant study using a subcutaneous pocket in 24 mice, and the investigators reported one case of extrusion but otherwise no change in weight or volume in the remaining 23 specimens. Dystrophic calcification and bone formation were also noted and, therefore, it is not an ideal candidate for soft tissue augmentation.[33] For the same reasons, Permacol™ might be better suited for abdominal reconstruction than breast reconstruction.

There are also concerns that the cross-linking process may prevent cellular ingrowth into the matrix, with experimental models demonstrating poor integration and intense local inflammation and foreign body reaction.[34,35] Non–cross-linked materials in a porcine model reportedly displayed earlier cell infiltration, extracellular matrix deposition, scaffold degradation, and neovascularization. These differences, however, diminished over time, suggesting other factors may be responsible.[36]

SURGIMEND® PRS (TEI BIOSCIENCES)

The only product derived from bovine tissue, SurgiMend®, was originally introduced for hernia repair and used neonatal tissue. SurgiMend® PRS was recently released in the past few years specifically for breast reconstruction and is composed of fetal bovine dermal collagen. TEI Biosciences selected this source to maximize the type III collagen, which is prominent in embryologic development and wound healing. The exact processing details are withheld as proprietary.

SurgiMend® Storage and Preparation

The inner pouch can be placed onto the sterile field. The SurgiMend® product is packaged dry, is stored at room temperature, comes in 2 thickness ranges (0.40–0.75 mm and 0.75–1.54 mm), and is available in large sheets up to 16 cm × 25 cm. SurgiMend® PRS is approximately 1 mm in thickness and available in smaller sizes, which are more appropriate for breast reconstruction. The unique feature of SurgiMend® PRS is fenestrations, which allow any fluid accumulation around the implant or expander to drain into the space underneath the mastectomy flaps and, theoretically, avoid the need to place a drain adjacent to the implant. It does require rehydration in room temperature saline for 60 seconds. No orientation is necessary and it is terminally sterile. SurgiMend® PRS should not be used in patients with sensitivity to collagen or bovine products.[37]

SurgiMend® Literature Reviews

The only report of SurgiMend® in the PubMed database discusses use in a staged nipple reconstruction to augment the thinned dermis with vascularized matrix. The investigators describe undermining a subdermal, supracapsular space at the future nipple reconstruction site and placing a disk of 2-mm thick SurgiMend® at the time of expander exchange. Four months later, a skate flap was elevated with the matrix, allowing for thicker flaps and histologic analysis–confirmed revascularization.[38]

ALLOMAX™ (BARD)

AlloMax™ is a sheet of human dermal collagen prepared using a trademarked Tutoplast process to remove all noncollagenous cellular components. Formerly marketed as NeoForm® (Mentor), AlloMax™ distinguishes itself as the only terminally sterilized human dermal graft. The Tutoplast process exposes the tissue to a series of 5 treatments starting with delipidization to remove lipids and red and white blood cells followed by an osmotic treatment to disrupt cell membranes to remove cellular components. An oxidative treatment removes immunogenic structures (ie, viruses) and then the solvent preserves the tissue matrix. Finally, a low dose of γ-irradiation ensures sterility.

AlloMax™ Storage and Preparation

The inner package is sterile and the matrix does not require orientation. It is available in 15 rectangular sizes and 1 square size, ranging from 2 cm × 4 cm to 16 cm × 20 cm. Unfortunately, only one thickness of the mesh is available and it ranges from 0.8 mm to 1.8 mm.

Contraindications for Use of AlloMax™

There are no absolute contraindications for use of AlloMax™.[39]

AlloMax™ Literature Reviews

AlloMax™ is directly referenced in only 2 citations in the PubMed database but in a study by Losken[40] using NeoForm®, involving 22 patients and 31 breast reconstructions, there were no cases of infection, foreign body reaction, seroma, or skin erythema. Histologic analysis in 2 random patients 3 months postoperatively showed vascular integration. In other studies, AlloMax™ was shown to have a high concentration of vascular endothelial growth factor and higher expression of interleukin-6 in an in vitro study.[14] The induction of monocytes and macrophages was also higher in AlloMax™ and FlexHD® than AlloDerm® but the clinical significance has yet to be determined.[41] AlloMax™ and AlloDerm® share many similar characteristics, as expected due to their similar tissue origins, but less inflammation at 4 weeks in a rat model for hernia repair.[42]

DERMACELL™ (LIFENET)

The most recently introduced product, DermACELL™, uses a patented LifeNet Health MATRACELL™ technology to create an acellular human dermal matrix. Similar to other ADMs, the tissue is not terminally sterile but has a sterility assurance level of 10^{-6}.

DermACELL™ Storage and Preparation

The product can be stored at room temperature and is fully hydrated and ready for use with an

Table 1
Summary of ADM characteristics

Product	Source	Prep Time	Prep	Refrigeration	Sterility	Orientation	Cross-linking	Shelf Life
AlloDerm®	Human	10–40 min	2 Baths of warm NS or LR	Yes/No[a]	No	Yes	No	2 y
AlloDerm® Ready to use	Human	2 min	Rinse in NS or LR	No	Yes	Yes	No	2 y
Strattice™	Porcine	2 min	Room-temp NS or LR	No	Yes	No	No	18 mo
DermaMatrix®	Human	<3 min	Room-temp NS or LR	No	No	Yes	No	3 y
FlexHD®	Human	None	None	No	No	Yes	No	3 y
Permacol™	Porcine	None	None	No	Yes	No	Yes	3 y
SurgiMend® PRS	Fetal bovine	60 s	Room-temp saline	No	Yes	No	No	3 y
AlloMax™	Human	3 min	Room-temp NS	No	Yes	No	No	5 y
DermACELL™	Human	None	None	No	No	Yes	No	2 y

Abbreviations: LR, lactated ringer's; NS, normal saline; Room-temp, room temperature.
[a] Alloderm before July 2010 required refrigeration.

inner package that is sterile. The package has a window through which the basement membrane side is visible for orientation. No rinse or rehydration is necessary before implantation. The available dimensions range from 2 cm × 2 cm to 6 cm × 16 cm and are available in 3 thicknesses (0.2–1.0 mm, 0.75–1.5 mm, and 1.25–2.0 mm).

DermACELL™ Contraindications for Use

DermACELL™ is exposed to gentamicin and vancomycin antibiotics during the aseptic process and, therefore, should be used with caution in patients with known sensitivities to these antibiotics.[43]

There are currently no published studies in the PubMed database regarding this product.

SUMMARY OF ADMs

The large array of ADMs available to reconstructive surgeons makes it challenging to understand the various distinctions and ultimately choose effectively. The clinical implications of the biologic source, processing, sterility, polarity, and other unknown factors have yet to be fully elucidated. A summary of these ADMs is provided in **Table 1**.

Inflammatory Response with ADMs

Most human dermal matrices require appropriate orientation during implantation. Generally this is easily distinguished but can cause problems if unrecognized. Failure to appropriately orient ADMs with a polarity can result in an inflammatory reaction, which mimics cellulitis with early erythema over the lower pole of the breast (superimposed over the anatomic extent of the acellular dermis). Clinically, there are no systemic signs of infection and there is no radiographic evidence of seroma or abscess. It is unclear if this is simply an inflammatory response to the tissue.[44] Some investigators have theorized that inadequate

Table 2
Comparison of ADM prices

	Calculated Approximate Price Per cm²
AlloDerm®	$28
Strattice™	$24.65–$30.76
DermaMatrix®	$28.51–$31.94
FlexHD®	$27.31–$34.76
Permacol™	$21.63
SurgiMend® PRS	$23
AlloMax™	$32.38
DermACELL™	$34

Note: Prices may vary across different institutions; for the most accurate information, contact a local sales representative. These data reflect the prices available to a single institution during an inquiry in August 2011. They do not reflect the charges to the patient and/or insurance.

Table 3
Summary of ADM advantages and disadvantages

	Advantages	Disadvantages
AlloDerm®	Well studied, recognized by insurance	Nonsterile pouch, long rehydration period, antibiotic sensitivity
Strattice™	Cost, sterile, short prep time, no orientation	Nonhuman, nonsterile pouch, short shelf life
DermaMatrix®	Short prep time, 4 thicknesses available	
FlexHD®	Ready to use	Cost
Permacol™	Cost, sterile, ready to use, no orientation	Nonhuman, cross-linking, odor, not for breast
SurgiMend® PRS	Cost, sterile, fenestrated, short prep time, no orientation	Nonhuman
AlloMax™	Only sterile human ADM, short prep time, long shelf life, no orientation	Cost
DermACELL™	Ready to use	Cost, antibiotic sensitivity

hydration or rinsing may contribute to the excess inflammatory response. An ADM without orientation would simplify the process and avoid possible complications.

Effect of ADM Preparation on Tissue

Several of these products are freeze-dried, which facilitates storage but must affect the tissue. Freeze-drying versus hydrated products in a rabbit hernia repair model did not show any difference in tensile strength, neovascularity, and adhesions but at 4 and 8 weeks, the hydrated dermal matrix demonstrated a reduced inflammatory response.[45] Perhaps hydrated ADMs are superior; certainly decreased operating room time wasted on rehydration is advantageous.

Infection Risk with ADMs

Logically, a terminally sterile ADM minimizes the risks of infection. This has been one of the primary concerns for surgeons reluctant to embrace ADMs for breast reconstruction. The use of ADMs may increase the odds of infection 5.37 times. These authors suggest that appropriate patient selection, modification of intraoperative technique, and postoperative care can minimize the risks.[6] A meta-analysis showed that the reported incidence of infection ranges from 0% to 8.9% with an overall rate of 5.2%.[46] Other studies, however, have found no significant difference.

An ideal ADM would be readily available without refrigeration; be contained within a sterile package; not require any rehydration or rinsing; have complete biocompatibility, a long shelf life, minimal inflammatory reaction, no contraindications, good long-term durability, and safety; be terminally sterile; be offered in multiple sizes with optimal thicknesses for tissue integration; be rapidly and maximally revascularized; not require orientation; and be available at a nominal cost.

ADM Costs

Most breast reconstruction costs are covered by insurance but because ADM use is considered experimental in some cases, product costs must be taken into account when selecting an implant. Some products have a fixed price based on area whereas other products vary. **Table 2** provides a comparison of costs.

Evaluation of New ADMs

As manufacturers continue to develop newer ADMs, it is critical to evaluate the advantages and disadvantages of each product with further clinical studies. Until then, breast surgeons must be aware of the advantages and disadvantages of each of these products (**Table 3**), discuss the options with each patient, and then select the appropriate ADM that most suits the needs of each individual patient.

REFERENCES

1. Nahabedian MY. AlloDerm performance in the setting of prosthetic breast surgery, infection, and irradiation. Plast Reconstr Surg 2009;124(6):1743–53.
2. Breuing KH, Colwell AS. Immediate breast tissue expander-implant reconstruction with inferolateral

AlloDerm hammock and postoperative radiation: a preliminary report. Eplasty 2009;9:e16.

3. Gamboa-Bobadilla GM. Implant breast reconstruction using acellular dermal matrix. Ann Plast Surg 2006;56(1):22–5.

4. Sbitany H, Sandeen SN, Amalfi AN, et al. Acellular dermis-assisted prosthetic breast reconstruction versus complete submuscular coverage: a head-to-head comparison of outcomes. Plast Reconstr Surg 2009;124(6):1735–40.

5. Spear SL, Seruya M, Clemens MW, et al. Acellular dermal matrix for the treatment and prevention of implant-associated breast deformities. Plast Reconstr Surg 2011;127(3):1047–58.

6. Chun YS, Verma K, Rosen H, et al. Implant-based breast reconstruction using acellular dermal matrix and the risk of postoperative complications. Plast Reconstr Surg 2010;125(2):429–36.

7. Parikh RP, Pappas-Politis E, Smith PD. Acellular dermal matrix masking detection of recurrent breast carcinoma: a novel complication. Aesthetic Plast Surg 2011.

8. Buck DW 2nd, Heyer K, Wayne JD, et al. Diagnostic dilemma: acellular dermis mimicking a breast mass after immediate tissue expander breast reconstruction. Plast Reconstr Surg 2009;124(1):174e–6e.

9. de Blacam C, Momoh AO, Colakoglu S, et al. Cost analysis of implant-based breast reconstruction with acellular dermal matrix. Ann Plast Surg 2011. [Epub ahead of print].

10. Breuing KH, Warren SM. Immediate bilateral breast reconstruction with implants and inferolateral AlloDerm slings. Ann Plast Surg 2005;55(3):232–9.

11. Bindingnavele V, Gaon M, Ota KS, et al. Use of acellular cadaveric dermis and tissue expansion in postmastectomy breast reconstruction. J Plast Reconstr Aesthet Surg 2007;60(11):1214–8.

12. Nahabedian MY. Secondary nipple reconstruction using local flaps and AlloDerm. Plast Reconstr Surg 2005;115(7):2056–61.

13. Garramone CE, Lam B. Use of AlloDerm in primary nipple reconstruction to improve long-term nipple projection. Plast Reconstr Surg 2007;119(6):1663–8.

14. LifeCell Corp. AlloDerm Regenerative Tissue Matrix. Available at: http://www.lifecell.com/alloderm-regenerative-tissue-matrix; http://www.lifecell.com/downloads/LC_Alloderm114_IFU_B_T4.pdf. Accessed August 20, 2011.

15. Sbitany H. Techniques to reduce seroma and infection in acellular dermis-assisted prosthetic breast reconstruction. Plast Reconstr Surg 2010;126(3):1121–2 [author reply: 1122].

16. Spear SL, Pelletiere CV, Lockwood M. Immediate breast reconstruction with tissue expanders and AlloDerm RTM. In: Spear SL, Wiley SC, Robb GL, et al, editors. Surgery of the breast: principles and art. 2nd edition. Philadelphia (PA): Lippincott Williams and Wilkins; 2006. p. 484–8.

17. Xu H, Wan H, Sandor M, et al. Host response to human acellular dermal matrix transplantation in a primate model of abdominal wall repair. Tissue Eng Part A 2008;14(12):2009–19.

18. Glasberg SB, D'Amico RA. Use of regenerative human acellular tissue (AlloDerm) to reconstruct the abdominal wall following pedicle TRAM flap breast reconstruction surgery. Plast Reconstr Surg 2006;118(1):8–15.

19. Salzberg CA, Ashikari AY, Koch RM, et al. An 8-year experience of direct-to-implant immediate breast reconstruction using human acellular dermal matrix (AlloDerm). Plast Reconstr Surg 2011;127(2):514–24.

20. Tran Cao HS, Tokin C, Konop J, et al. A preliminary report on the clinical experience with AlloDerm in breast reconstruction and its radiologic appearance. Am Surg 2010;76(10):1123–6.

21. Jansen LA, Macadam SA. The use of AlloDerm in postmastectomy alloplastic breast reconstruction: part I. A systematic review. Plast Reconstr Surg 2011;127(6):2232–44.

22. Jansen LA, Macadam SA. The use of AlloDerm in postmastectomy alloplastic breast reconstruction: part II. A cost analysis. Plast Reconstr Surg 2011;127(6):2245–54.

23. LifeCell Corp. Strattice Reconstructive Tissue Matrix. Available at: http://www.lifecell.com/strattice-reconstructive-tissue-matrix/255/; http://www.lifecell.com/downloads/StratticeIFU_T11.pdf. Accessed August 20, 2011.

24. Campbell KT, Burns NK, Rios CN, et al. Human versus non-cross-linked porcine acellular dermal matrix used for ventral hernia repair: comparison of in vivo fibrovascular remodeling and mechanical repair strength. Plast Reconstr Surg 2011;127(6):2321–32.

25. Katerinaki E, Zanetto U, Sterne GD. Histological appearance of Strattice tissue matrix used in breast reconstruction. J Plast Reconstr Aesthet Surg 2010;63(12):e840–1.

26. Synthes. DermaMatrix Acellular Dermis. Available at: http://www.synthes.com/sites/NA/Products/CMF/AcellularDermis/Pages/DermaMatrix_Acellular_Dermis.aspx; http://www.synthes.com/MediaBin/US%20DATA/Product%20Support%20Materials/Case%20Studies/CMF/MXCSBreastReconJ7731B.pdf. Accessed August 20, 2011.

27. Becker S, Saint-Cyr M, Wong C, et al. AlloDerm versus DermaMatrix in immediate expander-based breast reconstruction: a preliminary comparison of complication profiles and material compliance. Plast Reconstr Surg 2009;123(1):1–6 [discussion: 107–8].

28. Cole PD, Stal D, Sharabi SE, et al. A comparative, long-term assessment of four soft tissue substitutes. Aesthet Surg J 2011;31(6):674–81.

29. Ethicon. FlexHD Acellular Hydrated Dermis for Breast Reconstruction. Available at: http://www.ethicon360.com/products/flex-hd-acel-hydrated-dermis-breast-reconstruction; http://www.ethicon360.com/sites/default/files/products/PI%20_31-FLEX_HD_Derma_Matrix.pdf. Accessed August 20, 2011.

30. Eberli D, Rodriguez S, Atala A, et al. In vivo evaluation of acellular human dermis for abdominal wall repair. J Biomed Mater Res A 2010;93(4):1527–38.

31. Orenstein SB, Qiao Y, Kaur M, et al. Human monocyte activation by biologic and biodegradable meshes in vitro. Surg Endosc 2010;24(4):805–11.

32. Covidien. Permacol Surgical Implant. Available at: http://www.autosuture.com/autosuture/pagebuilder.aspx?topicID=170603&breadcrumbs=0:63659,30707:0,170596:0. Accessed August 20, 2011.

33. Kelley P, Gordley K, Higuera S, et al. Assessing the long-term retention and permanency of acellular cross-linked porcine dermal collagen as a soft-tissue substitute. Plast Reconstr Surg 2005;116(6):1780–4.

34. Jarman-Smith ML, Bodamyali T, Stevens C, et al. Porcine collagen crosslinking, degradation, and its capability for fibroblast adhesion and proliferation. J Mater Sci Mater Med 2004;15(8):925–32.

35. Petter-Puchner AH, Fortelny RH, Walder N, et al. Adverse effects associated with the use of porcine cross-linked collagen implants in an experimental model of incisional hernia repair. J Surg Res 2008;145(1):105–10.

36. Deeken CR, Melman L, Jenkins ED, et al. Histologic and biomechanical evaluation of crosslinked and non-crosslinked biologic meshes in a porcine model of ventral incisional hernia repair. J Am Coll Surg 2011;212(5):880–8.

37. TEI Biosciences. SurgiMend PRS for Plastic and Reconstructive Surgery. Available at: http://www.teibio.com/SurgiMend_PRS.aspx; http://www.teibio.com/Literature/SurgiMend/Product%20Information/Product%20Technology/PN%20606-999-022v00.pdf. Accessed August 20, 2011.

38. Craft RO, May JW Jr. Staged nipple reconstruction with vascularized SurgiMend acellular dermal matrix. Plast Reconstr Surg 2011;127(6):148e–9e.

39. Bard /Davol, Inc. AlloMax Breast Reconstruction. Available at: http://www.davol.com/products/soft-tissue-reconstruction/breast-reconstruction/biologics/allomax-breast-reconstruction/. Accessed August 20, 2011.

40. Losken A. Early results using sterilized acellular human dermis (Neoform) in post-mastectomy tissue expander breast reconstruction. Plast Reconstr Surg 2009. [Epub ahead of print].

41. Orenstein S, Qiao Y, Kaur M, et al. In vitro activation of human peripheral blood mononuclear cells induced by human biologic meshes. J Surg Res 2010;158(1):10–4.

42. Faleris JA, Hernandez RM, Wetzel D, et al. In-vivo and in-vitro histological evaluation of two commercially available acellular dermal matrices. Hernia 2011;15(2):147–56.

43. LifeNet Health. DermACELL. Available at: http://www.accesslifenethealth.org/classes/catalog/106. Accessed August 20, 2011.

44. Rawlani V, Buck DW 2nd, Johnson SA, et al. Tissue expander breast reconstruction using prehydrated human acellular dermis. Ann Plast Surg 2011;66(6):593–7.

45. Roth JS, Dexter DD, Lumpkins K, et al. Hydrated vs. freeze-dried human acellular dermal matrix for hernia repair: a comparison in a rabbit model. Hernia 2009;13(2):201–7.

46. Newman MI, Swartz KA, Samson MC, et al. The true incidence of near-term postoperative complications in prosthetic breast reconstruction utilizing human acellular dermal matrices: a meta-analysis. Aesthetic Plast Surg 2011;35(1):100–6.

Acellular Dermal Matrices in Breast Surgery: Tips and Pearls

Olubimpe A. Ayeni, MD, MPH, FRCSC,
Ahmed M.S. Ibrahim, MD, Samuel J. Lin, MD,
Sumner A. Slavin, MD*

KEYWORDS

- Acellular dermal matrices • Breast reconstruction
- Surgical techniques

Key Points

- Acellular dermal matrices (ADMs) are useful in primary prosthetic breast reconstruction as well as in the treatment of secondary deformities.
- A periareolar incision gives excellent access to the breast in secondary revision.
- When implanting ADMs, it is important to use a single, thick layer of the product.
- Patient selection is an important factor; in the postmastectomy setting, ADM-assisted reconstruction is appropriate in patients who have an adequate skin envelope.
- ADMs may alleviate the occurrence of complications by reducing the inflammatory changes that cause capsular contracture and capsule formation.
- One drawback to the use of ADMs is their cost.

Acellular dermal matrices (ADMs) have been used for postmastectomy breast reconstruction, primary and secondary breast augmentation, and reduction mammaplasty.[1,2] In postmastectomy breast reconstruction, ADMs can be used either to create an implant pocket in single-stage reconstruction or to create the inferolateral portion of the tissue expander pocket in 2-stage reconstruction. Specific deformities after cosmetic breast augmentation such as contour irregularities and implant malposition can be addressed with ADMs (**Table 1**).[1] The benefits of using ADMs include a low complication rate, the ability to provide needed tissue, and the ability to aid in repositioning the implant (**Table 2**). The disadvantages include the risk of infection and seroma, and high cost. The use of ADMs is a safe alternative for the correction of breast deformities after reconstructive and aesthetic breast surgery.

OVERVIEW OF ADMs IN BREAST SURGERY

ADMs became available in 1994 and the most commonly used ADMs in breast surgery are AlloDerm® (LifeCell, Branchburg, NJ, USA), Strattice™ (LifeCell Corporation, Branchburg, NJ, USA),

Disclosures: Dr Sumner Slavin is a LifeCell Consultant. None of the other authors have funding sources or conflicts of interest to disclose.
Division of Plastic Surgery, Beth Israel Deaconess Medical Center, Harvard Medical School, 110 Francis Street, Lowry Suite 5A, Boston, MA 02215, USA
* Corresponding author. Division of Plastic Surgery, 1101 Beacon Street, Brookline, MA 02446.
E-mail address: sslavin@bidmc.harvard.edu

Clin Plastic Surg 39 (2012) 177–186
doi:10.1016/j.cps.2012.02.003
0094-1298/12/$ – see front matter © 2012 Published by Elsevier Inc.

Table 1
Key technical considerations in using ADMs in breast surgery

| Reconstructive Breast Surgery | Aesthetic Breast Surgery | | Reduction Mammaplasty |
	Surface Irregularities	Implant Malposition	
ADM used to create implant pocket (single-stage reconstruction) or to cover inferolateral portion of the tissue expander (2-stage reconstruction) Used as a sling or hammock to anchor lower pole of pectoralis major Placed with dermal side facing mastectomy skin flaps Ensure mastectomy flaps are as thick as possible	Single layer of ADM placed between implant and overlying soft tissue Thick or ultrathick sheets most frequently used ADM placed in an onlay fashion ADM placed directly on capsule if no capsulotomy or capsulectomy required Parachuting technique aids in proper graft placement	ADM placed over areas of capsulorrhaphy and secured to the chest wall and capsule Dermal side oriented toward the capsule Avoid tension to prevent dimples and bands	Used as sling to support the inferior pedicle Plicate ADM in a horizontal fashion

DermaMatrix® (MTF/Synthes CMF, West Chester, PA, USA) and FlexHD® (Ethicon, New Brunswick, NJ, USA).

AlloDerm® regenerative tissue matrix is produced by removing the epidermis and cells from human cadaveric skin.[3] Strattice™ reconstructive tissue matrix (LifeCell Corp., Branchburg, NJ, USA) is derived from porcine dermis denuded of cells and sterilized using electron beam irradiation.[4] DermaMatrix® (MTF/Synthes CMF, West Chester, PA, USA) is human skin in which both the epidermis and dermis are removed from the

Table 2
Advantages of using ADMs in breast surgery

| Breast Reconstruction | Aesthetic Breast Surgery | | Reduction Mammaplasty |
	Surface Irregularities	Implant Malposition	
Provides soft tissue coverage over prosthesis Allows control of inframammary fold Permits creation of a larger implant pocket Decreases rate of capsular contracture Reduces time needed for entire reconstructive process Can expedite postoperative chemotherapy and radiation Decreases postoperative pain by limiting amount of dissection	Improved contour Minimizes the extent of dissection required	Prevents implant malposition in capsular contracture and symmastia Requires only a few tacking sutures	Better cosmetic outcome in terms of nipple-areola position and breast projection Lower risk of bottoming out

subcutaneous layer of tissue in a process using sodium chloride solution, rendering it sterile and preserving the original dermal collagen matrix.[5] FlexHD® acellular hydrated dermis is derived from donated human allograft skin.[6]

ADM Biomechanical Differences

A few biomechanical differences that are of clinical relevance exist between the various ADMs. AlloDerm® has been reported to have increased elasticity compared with DermaMatrix®[7] and Strattice™.[8] This quality is relevant in situations in which increased elasticity is preferred, such as in addressing capsular contracture, or when the goal is for the ADM to conform to the inferolateral curvature of the breast.[7] When the ADM is needed to provide support, such as in repositioning a displaced implant, a less elastic ADM like Strattice™ is preferred.[8] **Figs. 1–3** provide a comparison of the different biomechanical properties of various types of biologic meshes.

ADM Size

When deciding on the size of ADM to use, the patient is assessed preoperatively, and any surface irregularities or implant malposition are marked with the patient standing, sitting, lying down, and flexing the pectoralis major muscles. These markings aid in choosing the size of the ADM to be used.[1] Intraoperatively, the sheet of ADM is fashioned to the appropriate size of defect at the time of placement. With respect to the sizes of ADM to use, a 4-cm × 16-cm piece of AlloDerm®[9–11] is typically used; the thickness of ADM varies from 1.3 to 1.8 mm, and the thickness used depends on the indication. Spear and colleagues[12] devised a guideline for selection of

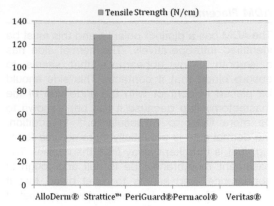

Fig. 2. A comparison of the tensile strength of different types of biologic mesh.

AlloDerm® size based on the arc length of the inframammary fold and the lateral mammary fold; for arc lengths of 18 cm or less, Spear and colleagues advocate a thick piece of 4 × 12 cm. For arc length greater than 18 cm, they advocate a thick piece of 4 × 16 cm.

ADM Preparation

In terms of preparation of the ADM, the matrix is hydrated in saline as instructed by the manufacturer. Different hydration times are required depending on the product; AlloDerm® requires at least 30 minutes of rehydration before its application[3] but DermaMatrix® can be rehydrated in 3 minutes.[5] It is important to examine the ADMs for dermal elements, such as hair, and to remove them if present. Sterile technique must be used when handling ADMs. The dermal matrix is handled by only 1 surgeon, after either changing or cleansing the gloves. The product is taken from the saline bath where it is soaking and placed directly in the wound so that it does not contact the operative field or the patient's skin.[13]

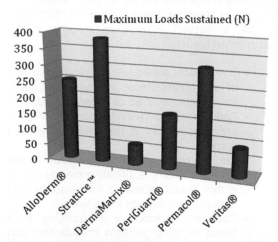

Fig. 1. A comparison of maximum loads sustained by different types of biologic mesh.

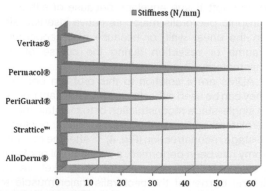

Fig. 3. A comparison of the stiffness of different types of biologic mesh.

ADM Placement

The ADM has a distinct polarity, and this must be identified intraoperatively. The dermal side has a smooth, shiny appearance that seems to absorb blood that it contacts. This side should be placed in contact with the underside of the mastectomy flap because it has been shown to be more likely to revascularize.[14] In addition, the dermal side is potentially more seroma forming, and is thus kept away from the implant. The basement membrane side is dull and rough in appearance, and seems to repel blood that it contacts. This side is placed down so that it contacts the implant.[13] It is important to avoid layering the ADM material because it is an avascular foreign body and this can increase the risk of infection and seroma formation.[1] For postoperative care, soft compression and a surgical bra postoperatively may be helpful in minimizing dead space.[13] Patients should remain on antibiotics to cover gram-positive skin flora for a 7-day period.

USES OF ADMs IN BREAST RECONSTRUCTION

Between one-half and two-thirds of women undergoing postmastectomy breast reconstruction choose alloplastic reconstruction, which makes prosthesis-based reconstruction the most common method of reconstruction in these patients.[15] After mastectomy, an implant[16] or a tissue expander is placed underneath the pectoralis major muscle, and the muscle covers the superior and medial poles of the prosthesis. The exposed inferior and lateral poles can be covered with subcutaneous tissue or by elevating serratus anterior or pectoralis minor muscles[17]; however, incomplete or inadequate coverage of the prosthesis can result in a higher risk of visible rippling, implant visibility or exposure, and contour irregularities.[7,11,14,18] Some patients have a deficiency of the soft tissue envelope because of either an atrophic pectoralis major, its native insertion site on the chest wall, or because of intraoperative trauma or resection during the course of the mastectomy.[19]

ADMs are a solution to this problem because they can be used either to create the implant pocket in single-stage reconstruction or to maintain the inferolateral portion of the tissue expander pocket in 2-stage reconstruction (**Fig. 4**).[20] After the mastectomy has been performed, a subpectoral pocket is developed. The boundaries of this pocket are the lateral border of the pectoralis major muscle to the second rib superiorly, the sternum medially, and the level of the contralateral inframammary fold inferiorly.[21] The inferior attachment of the pectoralis major muscle is dissected from the chest wall.[22]

Various techniques have been described to attach the ADM to local tissue. See **Box 1** for some technique tips for using ADMs in breast reconstruction.

Benefits of using ADMs in postmastectomy reconstruction include

- Providing soft tissue coverage over the prosthesis, especially when the skin flaps are deficient
- Allowing for control of the inframammary fold, permitting the creation of a larger implant pocket
- Decreasing the rate of capsular contracture.

These factors can potentially improve aesthetic outcomes.[10,20,21,25]

ADMs can also augment the perfusion of a vulnerable skin envelope[11] by offloading the mechanical stress caused by the implant weight on the skin envelope and the skin closure.[26]

Using ADMs can reduce the time needed for the entire reconstructive process by reducing the time or need for tissue expansion; in turn, this concept can expedite the start of adjuvant chemotherapy and radiation if needed. By limiting the amount of dissection during implant or expander placement, using ADMs may decrease postoperative pain.[25]

USES OF ADMs IN AESTHETIC BREAST SURGERY

Compared with the literature on postmastectomy reconstruction, there are fewer data on the uses of ADMs in cosmetic breast surgery. Despite this paucity of literature, there are unique challenges to be addressed in revision surgery of the augmented breast:

- The patients are frequently thin, have a lack of local breast tissue, and the breast envelope is often scarred or encapsulated.
- Patients tend to have high expectations and are disappointed in the need for revision surgery.
- Addressing 1 problem often leads to another; for example, plicating the capsule in a thin breast envelope can lead to skin dimpling and surface irregularities.
- Capsular excision or rearranging local tissue to cover surface irregularities can lead to an undesired change in the implant location.[1]

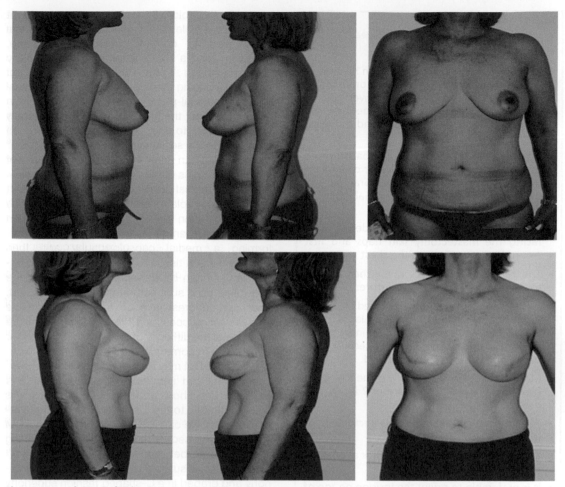

Fig. 4. Uses of ADMs for breast reconstruction after mastectomy (preoperative and postoperative).

Two categories of problems to correct with revision aesthetic breast surgery are surface irregularities and implant malposition.

USE OF ADMs TO CORRECT SURFACE IRREGULARITIES

Postoperative surface irregularities can include rippling or wrinkling, bulging, or capsular contracture.

Rippling is often an inherent feature of saline implants and is more obvious when the implant is covered with a thin soft tissue envelope.[27] In addition, tissue expansion often results in some degree of thinning of the overlying tissues, even with submuscular placement.[27]

- In patients who present with a focal area of tissue thinning with rippling or knuckling, a single layer of ADM can be placed between the implant and the overlying soft tissue for an improvement in contour (**Fig. 5**).

- A periareolar incision provides excellent exposure and limits the amount of additional incisions. Thick or ultrathick sheets are most frequently used.
- The dermal side of the graft is placed in contact with the capsule in an onlay fashion and secured with absorbable sutures at the corners; placement of the grafts in an onlay fashion minimizes the extent of dissection required.[24] In this setting, the ADM is used as a tissue-thickener for camouflaging implant visibility.
- In addition, the ADM can be laid directly on the capsule if no capsulotomy or capsulectomy is needed. A parachuting[1,12] technique often aids in placing the graft in the correct location.

ADMs Versus Fat Grafting

Although autologous fat injections are gaining popularity as a method of correcting contour

---

Box 1
Technique tips for using ADM in breast reconstruction

- An ADM sling[11] or hammock[23] can be used to anchor the lower pole of the pectoralis major muscle by attaching it to the lower pole of the released pectoralis major superiorly, the serratus anterior flap laterally, and the chest wall inferomedially.

- After irrigating the pocket with bacitracin in sterile saline, the tissue expander or implant is then placed in the subpectoral pocket, covering the superior and medial poles of the prosthesis.

- The ADM is placed with the dermal side facing the mastectomy skin flaps and first secured by suturing it to the chest wall.

- The free edge of the pectoralis is then sutured to the ADM with a running suture.

- Two closed-suction drains are placed below the mastectomy skin flaps; 1 drain is placed in the axilla because this area tends to drain moderate amounts in most cases[13] and the second drain runs along the inframammary fold.

- Mastectomy skin flaps are trimmed to yield bleeding margins for closure in 2 layers and dressed.[22]

- Tension-free closure of the mastectomy flaps is crucial.

- Ensuring that the flaps are as thick as possible is also important.

- It is preferable to orient the incision on top of the muscle as opposed to directly over the ADM.

- Because textured implants can cause noticeable rippling,[24] these implants are to be avoided.

---

deformities, compared with ADMs they have several disadvantages:

- Fat grafting has a high resorption rate
- Fat grafting requires a donor site
- Fat grafting can result in complications such as calcifications, cyst formation, infection, and induration.[28]

In addition, long-term data of fat grafting to the native breast are lacking. There are early reports that are now evaluating the impact of breast cancer surveillance with fat grafting.

USE OF ADMs TO CORRECT IMPLANT MALPOSITION

Implant malposition can occur as a result of capsular contracture or with malposition of the inframammary fold with or without bottoming out of the lower pole.[29] A variety of methods have been used to correct capsular contracture, including using a combination of capsulorrhaphy and marionette sutures.[9,29] Another method involves changing the implant pocket from a subglandular to dual-plane position with the addition of an ADM graft; the graft is fixed to the pectoralis major muscle, to the perichondrium of the rib cage, and to the serratus anterior muscle flap.[29,30]

Symmastia can result from excessive release of the medial origins of the pectoralis major muscles, resulting in medial displacement of the implants. It occurs when implants are placed too close to the midline or when an iatrogenic communication occurs. One management option involves performing a medial capsulorrhaphy and then suturing the soft tissue to the sternum. The posterior capsule can be dissected from the rib cage and rolled up if subpectoral implants were used. These procedures have been met with variable degrees of success and are prone to failure because of the difficulty of separating the capsular pockets.[31] To correct implant malposition in symmastia, the ADM may be placed over areas of capsulorrhaphy and secured to the chest wall and capsule: the short edge of the AlloDerm® is sutured directly to the displaced fold and then redraped over the capsule of the breast.[32] An ADM can also be used as a medial, C-shaped sling that is created between the 2 implants.[31] A graft of AlloDerm® is sutured to the rib periosteum inferiorly and draped in a C-shaped fashion superiorly to the anterior capsule.[31]

ADMs are secured with 3.0 Vicryl (Ethicon Inc, Somerville, NJ, USA) or Monocryl (Ethicon Inc, Somerville, NJ, USA). Only a few tacking sutures are needed in most cases; however, in the correction of symmastia, more sutures may be required to secure the ADM and avoid permanent suture dimpling of the skin. Tension should be avoided because surface dimples and bands can occur.

USE OF ADMs IN REDUCTION MAMMAPLASTY

A common postoperative finding in inferior pedicle breast reduction is an upward rotation of the nipple-areola complex and descent of the breast parenchyma, otherwise called star-gazing or bottoming out. This finding occurs because of recurrent skin laxity. In attempting to address this issue, Brown and colleagues[2] devised an approach in which AlloDerm® could be used as a sling to support the inferior pedicle and hence prevent this unwanted breast deformity. These investigators describe using an ADM as an

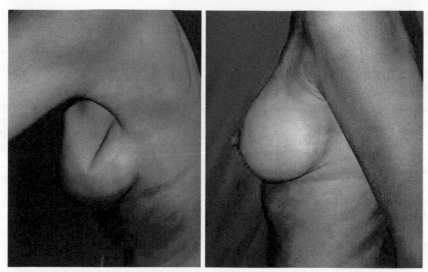

Fig. 5. Use of ADMs for secondary deformities in breast reconstruction (preoperative and postoperative).

"internal brassiere" for support of the pedicle. To help gain a better cosmetic outcome in terms of nipple-areola position and breast projection, the pedicle superior to the ADM was plicated in a horizontal fashion in addition to suturing AlloDerm® to the chest wall as a sling. In the postoperative period, no nipple loss was noted, and 2 patients developed complications; 1 had partial flap necrosis and the other had cellulitis. No bottoming out was seen in any of the patients.

COMPLICATIONS WITH ADMs

The use of ADMs does not seem to significantly increase the risk of postoperative complications[33] but is not without risk.

Microbial Contamination

AlloDerm® is the most widely used ADM product, and when tested to confirm the absence of microbial contamination, it is not terminally sterile.[17] Because AlloDerm® comes from a human donor, there is a risk of transmitting communicable diseases such as viral hepatitis and human immunodeficiency virus (although there have been no such reported cases). The product meets the standards of tissue banking and donor screening established by the American Association of Tissue Banking and the US Food and Drug Administration.[1]

Infection

In the last few years, studies have been published that compare the complication rates of postmastectomy reconstruction using prostheses with or without AlloDerm®. Only 1 of these studies[34] reported a statistically significant increase in infection and 1 study reported an increased seroma rate in the AlloDerm® group.[17] As ADM recellularizes, revascularizes, and becomes incorporated into the host tissue, it has the potential to overcome infection. However, it takes time for the ADM to recellularize and revascularize, providing a window in which infection can occur.[35] In an animal model, Eppley[36] observed that rolled or multilayered ADM revascularized more slowly or, in some areas, not at all when compared with a single flat sheet of ADM. This finding indicates that potential rolling or bunching of ADM can lead to poor vascularization, with an increased risk of infection.[36] When the ADM comes in contact with the nipple-areola complex, it may be exposed to contamination from *Staphylococcus* species, which can be abundant in the distal mammary ducts. Therefore, it is best to avoid ADM placement in this region.[1]

Radiation Tolerance

There is ongoing debate about the ability of ADMs to tolerate exposure to radiation. Studies that have compared complications in irradiated and nonirradiated breasts have indicated a higher rate of complications in irradiated versus nonirradiated breasts.

- Spear and colleagues[12] observed an 11-fold higher rate of total complications in irradiated versus nonirradiated breasts (45.5% vs 4.3%) after ADM-assisted tissue expander/implant reconstruction.
- Salzberg and colleagues[21] noted a 4-fold higher rate of complications in irradiated versus nonirradiated breasts.

- Nahabedian[8] reported a higher incidence of infection (8.3% vs 3.9%), incisional dehiscence (13.0% vs 1.3%), and seroma (13.0% vs 2.6%) in ADM-assisted implant-based irradiated versus nonirradiated breasts.

However, overall, the risk of infection did not vary with or without AlloDerm®.

Rawlani and colleagues[37] found that the overall complication rate in irradiated breasts was 30.8% (compared with 13.7% in nonirradiated breasts, $P = .0749$). Despite this higher rate of complications, ADM-assisted tissue expander reconstruction seems to resist radiation effects more than plain tissue expander reconstructions,[12,37,38] or at least have a similar rate of complications.[19]

Diagnostic Dilemmas

There has been a report of a potential diagnostic dilemma, with ADM mimicking a new breast mass in a patient who had had a previous mastectomy.[39] ADMs can undergo reactive inflammatory changes and be confused as masses within the breast, especially with the minimal subcutaneous fat in this area and with thin mastectomy skin flaps. Patients should be informed that ADM use in breast surgery can lead to induration, palpable scarring, and the potential need for further diagnostic studies.[39] With the sophisticated imaging available, it seems that the appearance of ADMs is different from and does not mask recurrences on either a mammogram or a magnetic resonance imaging scan of the breast.[40]

OUTCOMES WITH ADMs

In a retrospective study by Hartzell and colleagues,[1] a single surgeon's experience using ADMs after breast augmentation from 2005 to 2009 was analyzed:

- Twenty-three patients (38 breasts) were included
- Implant malposition was reported in 22 breasts
- Surface irregularities were reported in 28 breasts
- Malposition and surface regularities combined appeared in 12 patients.

After their revision procedures using an ADM

- Twenty patients showed improvement in the aesthetic appearance of their breasts
- Three patients required an additional procedure

- One patient developed an infection and the ADM was removed.

In 78 consecutive patients who underwent revisionary breast augmentation/mastopexies with ADM

- All patients had their implant-related complications successfully corrected by a site change and the use of an ADM.[38]
- No capsular contractures were reported.
- There were 2 complications: implant malposition and hematoma formation.

These data suggest that, with the use of ADMs, the capsular contracture rate after secondary augmentation and augmentation mastopexy procedures may be reduced.[38]

Basu and colleagues[41] found that when compared with native breast capsules, ADM had lower levels of inflammatory parameters:

- Capsule fibrosis
- Vessel proliferation
- Granulation tissue formation
- Fibroblast cellularity
- Chronic inflammatory changes
- Foreign body giant cell inflammatory reaction.

AlloDerm® decreases radiation-related inflammation and delays or diminishes pseudoepithelium formation and thus may slow progression of capsular formation, fibrosis, and contraction.[42] These findings suggest that ADM may show certain properties that may reduce formation of a capsule and therefore provide an alternative to total submuscular implant placement in breast reconstruction procedures.[41,43]

Costs of ADMs

One of the drawbacks to the use of ADMs is their cost. A 6-cm × 16-cm thick AlloDerm® sheet cost $3463 (USD) per sheet as of January 2010 (Jansen; economic analysis).[44] However, direct-to-implant reconstruction with AlloDerm® was found to be less expensive than 2-stage non-AlloDerm® reconstruction.[44] Strattice™ is less expensive than AlloDerm®. In addition, Strattice™ is available in specific sizes and shapes to reduce cost and minimize waste.[8]

SUMMARY

ADMs have many applications in breast surgery. In addition to postmastectomy breast reconstruction, ADMs may be safe to use with a limited number of complications in the setting of contour deformities after cosmetic breast operations. The 1 drawback is that they are expensive.[44] The use of ADMs is a safe alternative for the correction of breast deformities after reconstructive and aesthetic surgery. Appropriate patient selection, operative technique, and postoperative management are crucial in successful application of ADMs to breast surgery.

REFERENCES

1. Hartzell TL, Taghinia AH, Chang J, et al. The use of human acellular dermal matrix for the correction of secondary deformities after breast augmentation: results and costs. Plast Reconstr Surg 2010; 126(5):1711–20.
2. Brown RH, Izaddoost S, Bullocks JM. Preventing the "bottoming out" and "star-gazing" phenomena in inferior pedicle breast reduction with an acellular dermal matrix internal brassiere. Aesthetic Plast Surg 2010;34(6):760–7.
3. LifeCell. Breast reconstruction. 2011. Available at: http://www.lifecell.com/strattice-reconstructive-tissue-matrix/255/. Accessed December 7, 2011.
4. LifeCell. KCI's LifeCell Granted CE Mark for its Strattice(R) Reconstructive Tissue Matrix. 2008. Available at: http://www.kci1.com/cs/Satellite?c=KCI_News_C&childpagename=KCI%2FKCILayout&cid=1229631881542&pagename=KCI1Wrapper. Accessed December 7, 2011.
5. Synthes. DermaMatrix Acellular Dermis. Human dermal collagen matrix. 2006. Available at: http://www.synthes.com/MediaBin/US%20DATA/Product%20Support%20Materials/Brochures/CMF/MXBRODermaMatrixAcellular-J7237D.pdf. Accessed December 7, 2011.
6. MTF. FlexHD Acellular Hydrated Dermis. 2006. Available at: http://www.mtf.org/professional/flex_hd.html. Accessed December 7, 2011.
7. Becker S, Saint-Cyr M, Wong C, et al. AlloDerm versus DermaMatrix in immediate expander-based breast reconstruction: a preliminary comparison of complication profiles and material compliance. Plast Reconstr Surg 2009;123(1):1–6 [discussion: 107–8].
8. Nahabedian MY. AlloDerm performance in the setting of prosthetic breast surgery, infection, and irradiation. Plast Reconstr Surg 2009;124(6): 1743–53.
9. Breuing KH, Warren SM. Immediate bilateral breast reconstruction with implants and inferolateral AlloDerm slings. Ann Plast Surg 2005;55(3):232–9.
10. Gamboa-Bobadilla GM. Implant breast reconstruction using acellular dermal matrix. Ann Plast Surg 2006;56(1):22–5.
11. Zienowicz RJ, Karacaoglu E. Implant-based breast reconstruction with allograft. Plast Reconstr Surg 2007;120(2):373–81.

12. Spear SL, Parikh PM, Reisin E, et al. Acellular dermis-assisted breast reconstruction. Aesthetic Plast Surg 2008;32(3):418–25.
13. Sbitany H. Techniques to reduce seroma and infection in acellular dermis-assisted prosthetic breast reconstruction. Plast Reconstr Surg 2010;126(3): 1121–2 [author reply: 1122].
14. Namnoum JD. Expander/implant reconstruction with AlloDerm: recent experience. Plast Reconstr Surg 2009;124(2):387–94.
15. Le GM, O'Malley CD, Glaser SL, et al. Breast implants following mastectomy in women with early-stage breast cancer: prevalence and impact on survival. Breast Cancer Res 2005;7(2):R184–93.
16. Askari M, Cohen MJ, Grossman PH, et al. The use of acellular dermal matrix in release of burn contracture scars in the hand. Plast Reconstr Surg 2011; 127(4):1593–9.
17. Liu AS, Kao HK, Reish RG, et al. Postoperative complications in prosthesis-based breast reconstruction using acellular dermal matrix. Plast Reconstr Surg 2011;127(5):1755–62.
18. Colwell AS, Breuing KH. Improving shape and symmetry in mastopexy with autologous or cadaveric dermal slings. Ann Plast Surg 2008; 61(2):138–42.
19. Bindingnavele V, Gaon M, Ota KS, et al. Use of acellular cadaveric dermis and tissue expansion in postmastectomy breast reconstruction. J Plast Reconstr Aesthet Surg 2007;60(11):1214–8.
20. Jansen LA, Macadam SA. The use of AlloDerm in postmastectomy alloplastic breast reconstruction: part I. A systematic review. Plast Reconstr Surg 2011;127(6):2232–44.
21. Salzberg CA, Ashikari AY, Koch RM, et al. An 8-year experience of direct-to-implant immediate breast reconstruction using human acellular dermal matrix (AlloDerm). Plast Reconstr Surg 2011;127(2): 514–24.
22. Lanier ST, Wang ED, Chen JJ, et al. The effect of acellular dermal matrix use on complication rates in tissue expander/implant breast reconstruction. Ann Plast Surg 2010;64(5):674–8.
23. Breuing KH, Colwell AS. Inferolateral AlloDerm hammock for implant coverage in breast reconstruction. Ann Plast Surg 2007;59(3):250–5.
24. Duncan DI. Correction of implant rippling using allograft dermis. Aesthet Surg J 2001;21(1):81–4.
25. Topol BM, Dalton EF, Ponn T, et al. Immediate single-stage breast reconstruction using implants and human acellular dermal tissue matrix with adjustment of the lower pole of the breast to reduce unwanted lift. Ann Plast Surg 2008;61(5):494–9.
26. Liao EC, Breuing KH. Breast mound salvage using vacuum-assisted closure device as bridge to reconstruction with inferolateral AlloDerm hammock. Ann Plast Surg 2007;59(2):218–24.

27. Baxter RA. Intracapsular allogenic dermal grafts for breast implant-related problems. Plast Reconstr Surg 2003;112(6):1692–6 [discussion: 1697–8].

28. Hyakusoku H, Ogawa R, Ono S, et al. Complications after autologous fat injection to the breast. Plast Reconstr Surg 2009;123(1):360–70 [discussion: 371–2].

29. Spear SL, Seruya M, Clemens MW, et al. Acellular dermal matrix for the treatment and prevention of implant-associated breast deformities. Plast Reconstr Surg 2011;127(3):1047–58.

30. Mofid MM, Singh NK. Pocket conversion made easy: a simple technique using alloderm to convert subglandular breast implants to the dual-plane position. Aesthet Surg J 2009;29(1):12–8.

31. Curtis MS, Mahmood F, Nguyen MD, et al. Use of AlloDerm for correction of symmastia. Plast Reconstr Surg 2010;126(4):192e–3e.

32. Nahabedian MY. Discussion. The use of human acellular dermal matrix for the correction of secondary deformities after breast augmentation: results and costs. Plast Reconstr Surg 2010;126(5):1721–2.

33. Preminger BA, McCarthy CM, Hu QY, et al. The influence of AlloDerm on expander dynamics and complications in the setting of immediate tissue expander/implant reconstruction: a matched-cohort study. Ann Plast Surg 2008;60(5):510–3.

34. Chun YS, Verma K, Rosen H, et al. Implant-based breast reconstruction using acellular dermal matrix and the risk of postoperative complications. Plast Reconstr Surg 2010;125(2):429–36.

35. Isken T, Onyedi M, Izmirli H, et al. Abdominal fascial flaps for providing total implant coverage in one-stage breast reconstruction: an autologous solution. Aesthetic Plast Surg 2009;33(6):853–8.

36. Eppley BL. Experimental assessment of the revascularization of acellular human dermis for soft-tissue augmentation. Plast Reconstr Surg 2001; 107(3):757–62.

37. Rawlani V, Buck DW 2nd, Johnson SA, et al. Tissue expander breast reconstruction using prehydrated human acellular dermis. Ann Plast Surg 2011; 66(6):593–7.

38. Maxwell GP, Gabriel A. Use of the acellular dermal matrix in revisionary aesthetic breast surgery. Aesthet Surg J 2009;29(6):485–93.

39. Buck DW 2nd, Heyer K, Wayne JD, et al. Diagnostic dilemma: acellular dermis mimicking a breast mass after immediate tissue expander breast reconstruction. Plast Reconstr Surg 2009;124(1):174e–6e.

40. Tran Cao HS, Tokin C, Konop J, et al. A preliminary report on the clinical experience with AlloDerm in breast reconstruction and its radiologic appearance. Am Surg 2010;76(10):1123–6.

41. Basu CB, Leong M, Hicks MJ. Acellular cadaveric dermis decreases the inflammatory response in capsule formation in reconstructive breast surgery. Plast Reconstr Surg 2010;126(6):1842–7.

42. Komorowska-Timek E, Oberg KC, Timek TA, et al. The effect of AlloDerm envelopes on periprosthetic capsule formation with and without radiation. Plast Reconstr Surg 2009;123(3):807–16.

43. Salzberg CA. Nonexpansive immediate breast reconstruction using human acellular tissue matrix graft (AlloDerm). Ann Plast Surg 2006;57(1):1–5.

44. Jansen LA, Macadam SA. The use of AlloDerm in postmastectomy alloplastic breast reconstruction: part II. A cost analysis. Plast Reconstr Surg 2011; 127(6):2245–54.

Acellular Dermal Matrices: Economic Considerations in Reconstructive and Aesthetic Breast Surgery

Sheina A. Macadam, MD, MHS, FRCSC*, Peter A. Lennox, MD, FRCSC

KEYWORDS

- Acellular dermal matrices • Economic analysis
- Breast reconstruction • Breast aesthetic surgery

Key Points

- A formal cost evaluation of the use of ADMs in breast surgery requires knowledge of the cost of the product, the cost of the surgery being performed, the cost of potential outcomes, costs of patient time expended for the intervention, costs associated with care giving, economic costs borne by employers, and costs borne by the rest of society.

- A true cost-utility analysis of the use of ADM in breast surgery requires high quality outcomes studies and standardized health utility states which are currently lacking from the literature.

- Preliminary cost minimization analysis in a Canadian center shows that conversion of traditional 2-stage total submuscular alloplastic reconstruction to 1-stage alloplastic reconstruction using ADM results in cost savings as a result of elimination of the cost of the tissue expander and second-stage surgery.

- On short-term follow-up, addition of ADMs to alloplastic breast reconstruction (1-stage and 2-stage outcomes combined) seems to result in favorable outcomes for capsular contracture, late revision, and total implant loss compared with traditional 2-stage reconstruction. Rates of mastectomy flap necrosis, seroma, and infection are slightly higher than those seen in the Allergan and Mentor core studies for two-stage non-ADM reconstruction.

- In the setting of aesthetic surgery ADMs may prove cost-effective if a decreased subsequent revision rate with use of ADM at the first revision surgery can be proven.

The cost of introducing a new device into surgical practice needs to be evaluated when there is uncertainty as to whether there is an improved outcome with the new technique. If the new device is more expensive than the standard alternative, medical administrators require decision-analytical data to illustrate improvement in patient outcomes to justify the additional cost.

Similarly, if outcomes are the same, but a new device lowers the cost of patient care, well-collected data illustrating the cost savings are essential (**Fig. 1**).

Economic analyses in surgery are required to show the relative benefits of a new or alternative intervention. The use of autologous dermal grafts in breast reconstructive surgery has been described

---

Financial Disclosure: Dr Lennox is a speaker for LifeCell. No funding was obtained for the preparation of this manuscript.

Division of Plastic & Reconstructive Surgery, University of British Columbia and Vancouver General Hospital, 2nd Floor, JPP 2. 855 West, 12th Avenue, Vancouver, BC V5Z 1M9, Canada
* Corresponding author. 1000-777 West Broadway, Vancouver, BC V5Z4J7, Canada.
E-mail address: drsamacadam@gmail.com

Clin Plastic Surg 39 (2012) 187–216
doi:10.1016/j.cps.2012.02.007

plasticsurgery.theclinics.com

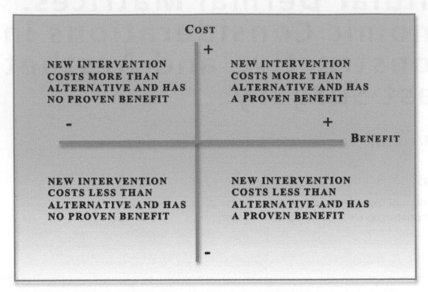

Fig. 1. Cost-benefit analysis for introduction of a new surgical intervention.

since 1979.[1,2] Because of variability in revascularization and donor site morbidity, acellular dermal matrices (ADMs) were developed. ADMs have shown promise for use in both aesthetic and reconstructive breast surgery, but concerns about their use remain because of the significant costs associated with these products.

ECONOMIC ANALYSIS IN SURGICAL LITERATURE

The use of ADMs in breast surgery is relatively new. Since 2001, there have been 27 published series outlining surgical technique and preliminary outcomes in patients undergoing breast reconstruction[3–29] and 9 series describing the use of ADMs in aesthetic breast surgery (**Tables 1** and **2**).[30–38] One formal meta-analysis, 1 systematic review, and 2 cost analyses have been published (see **Table 1**).[39–42]

Economic evaluation in the surgical literature is rare. A systematic review of the number of published cost-utility studies over a 6-year period revealed 649 publications in the medical literature compared with 57 in the surgical literature.[43] These investigators state: "the lack of formal economic evaluation in the surgical literature likely stems from the complexity of the subject and (with few exceptions) the lack of surgeon training in clinical research methodology."[43] In current health care systems, surgeons should make decisions based not only on patient outcomes but also on the cost of a particular surgical intervention. Cost analysis allows for comparison of costs of competing medical interventions and their corresponding health outcomes states.[44,45] Such analyses can

aid health policy decision makers in weighing the benefits and risks of a new surgical technique and to decide whether the benefits provided by a new procedure warrant potential additional costs.

Four different types of economic evaluation are used in the medical literature[46–49]:

1. Cost-minimization analysis
2. Cost-effectiveness analysis
3. Cost-utility analysis
4. Cost-benefit analysis.

Cost-minimization analysis is used to compare 2 alternatives that have comparable outcomes but different costs. In this type of analysis, cost in dollars is the only reported metric.

A cost-effectiveness analysis reports outcomes in physical units, such as lives saved or successful surgeries or cost per outcome.

A cost-utility analysis is similar to the cost-effectiveness analysis, but reports outcomes in cost per quality-adjusted life-year (QALY). A QALY is a value determined by the number of extended life-years in a particular health (utility) state attributable to a particular intervention, in which the utility is the preference of an individual or society for the health state.[46]

A cost-benefit analysis attaches a value to the cost-effectiveness of an intervention by asking health care consumers what they would be willing to pay for a certain health outcome.

The use of ADM in breast surgery is relatively new, with the first reports published in 2001 and 2003.[30,34] Because of its relative newness in breast surgery, utilities for health states in patients who have had breast surgery living with and without

ADM have not been standardized. A formal cost-utility analysis adhering to the guidelines set out by the Panel on Cost-Effectiveness in Health and Medicine comparing breast surgery (aesthetic and reconstructive) with and without the use of ADM is therefore difficult.[50] Only 2 studies have been published that have evaluated the cost of implementation of ADM into breast surgery.[41,42] Jansen's cost-minimization analysis compared traditional 2-stage tissue expander/implant breast reconstruction with 1-stage breast reconstruction using ADM. Outcomes were estimated from a previous systematic review.[40] De Blacam's cost-minimization analysis compared 2-stage tissue expander/implant reconstruction, 1-stage reconstruction using ADM, and 2-stage tissue expander/implant reconstruction using ADM. Outcomes were estimated from weighted averages from a literature review.[42] Inherent limitations of this type of cost analysis include the variability in reporting of the included articles. The probabilities of clinically relevant outcomes after breast surgery using ADMs are difficult to estimate because all published studies have been case series, the largest including 260 patients who had had single-stage breast reconstruction.[24] Ideally, outcome probabilities should be estimated from an average of results from several high-quality studies.

DEVELOPMENT OF ADM USE IN BREAST SURGERY

ADMs have been used successfully across multiple specialties and for varied applications including the resurfacing of burn injuries, gingival recession, abdominal hernia repair, aesthetic facial contouring, eyelid reconstruction, tympanic membrane reconstruction, and dural replacement.[51–58]

In 2001, the first report of ADM (AlloDerm®, Life-Cell Corporation, Branchburg, NJ, USA) use was documented in aesthetic breast surgery in a series of 34 patients with surface irregularities after breast augmentation.[34] Applications in this field expanded to include correction of symmastia, implant malposition, and capsular atrophy.[30]

In 2005, Breuing and Warren[8] reported the first use of an ADM in breast reconstruction. In their series, 10 patients underwent bilateral mastectomy with immediate reconstruction using an implant and inferior AlloDerm® sling. This series marked the introduction of ADM-assisted single-stage breast reconstruction. Benefits of ADM use in single-stage breast reconstruction such as improved lower pole projection, additional implant coverage, and maximization of the breast skin envelope in immediate reconstruction were soon recognized, and in 2007 Bindingnavele and colleagues[7] reported the first series of patients to undergo 2-stage reconstruction with AlloDerm®. Purported benefits of this application include decreased postoperative pain, expedited expansion, and elimination of elevation of the serratus anterior lateral muscle sling. Use of ADM in breast reconstruction surgery evolved from the initial applications in breast aesthetic surgery and has now become a standard option in alloplastic reconstructive surgery.

ADM Products Expanding

Since these early reports, ADM use in breast reconstructive and aesthetic surgery has become common. The introduction of human-derived Allo-Derm to the ADM market in 1994 was followed by development of ADMs from both allogenic and xenogenic sources. The most commonly used and studied matrix is AlloDerm®, but recently developed products including FlexHD® (Ethicon [Johnson & Johnson], San Angelo, TX, USA), DermaMatrix® (Synthes, Inc., West Chester, PA, USA), AlloMax™ (Davol, A BARD Company, Warwick, RI, USA), SurgiMend® (TEI Biosciences, Boston, MA, USA), and Strattice™ (LifeCell Corporation, Branchburg, NJ, USA) are now being used for the same breast-related indications. Each product differs in terms of source, shelf life, rehydration time, sterility, and cost.

Advantages and Disadvantages

Increased surgeon awareness, perceived benefits, and early favorable results fuel the demand for ADM by patients undergoing breast surgery. Steady surgical procedure volumes continue to support demand for the use of these products. However, the potential advantages must be weighed against the increased costs. Budgetary concerns among health care facilities may lead to pressure on companies to lower product pricing or to negotiate discounts on single items as well as bundled product purchases to curb costs. This situation may offset part of the added cost of these products, but as usage gains momentum it is necessary for surgeons to complete rigorous assessment of outcomes to support the common perception that ADM use in breast surgery decreases the need for revisional surgery and thus may prove cost-effective.

SCIENTIFIC CONSIDERATIONS IN USE OF ADMs IN BREAST RECONSTRUCTION

Biocompatible dermal matrices are produced from allogenic and xenogenic sources by removal of the epidermis and all of the cells of the dermis. The most extensively studied ADM that has been used

Table 1
(continued)

Author, Location	Title	Journal	Year	Sample Size	1-Stage vs 2-Stage	Sample Population	Design	Surgical Technique
Derderian et al,[12] United States	Wise-pattern breast reconstruction modification using AlloDerm® and a vascularized dermal-subcutaneous pedicle	Ann Plast Surg	2009	20 patients	1-stage Immediate	Mean age: N/D 5 patients radiated preoperatively	RCS	Standard with variable SA elevation for lateral implant coverage
Ellsworth et al,[13] United States	Breast implant salvage with the use of acellular dermal matrix after partial mastectomy	Plast Reconstr Surg	2010	1 patient	1-stage	Age: 60 y Previous bilateral subglandular augmentation with right-sided breast cancer Postreconstruction radiation	Case report	AlloDerm® used to reinforce lateral capsule
Gamboa-Bobadilla,[14] United States	Implant breast reconstruction using ADM	Ann Plast Surg	2006	11 patients, 13 breasts	1-stage Immediate and delayed	Median age: 58 y (range: 41–68 y)	RCS	Standard
Jansen & Macadam,[40] Canada	The use of AlloDerm® in postmastectomy alloplastic breast reconstruction: Part I. A systematic review	Plast Reconstr Surg	2011	N/A	1-stage	N/A	Systematic review	N/A
Jansen & Macadam,[41] Canada	The use of AlloDerm® in postmastectomy alloplastic breast reconstruction: Part II. A cost analysis	Plast Reconstr Surg	2011	N/A	N/A	N/A	Cost analysis	N/A

Lanier et al,[15] United States	The effect of ADM use on complication rates in tissue expander/implant breast reconstruction	Ann Plast Surg	2010	75 patients ADM group 52 patients non-ADM group	2-stage Immediate	Mean age: 51 y	RCS	Standard
Liu et al,[16] United States	Postoperative complications in prosthesis-based breast reconstruction using ADM	Plast Reconstr Surg	2011	192 patients, 266 breasts	1-stage 2-stage Immediate	N/D	RCS	Standard
Losken,[17] United States	Early results using sterilized ADM (neoform) in postmastectomy tissue expander breast reconstruction	Plast Reconstr Surg	2009	22 patients, 31 breasts	2-stage Immediate	Mean age: 48 y	PCS	Standard
Margulies et al,[18] United States	Total skin-sparing mastectomy without preservation of the nipple-areola complex	Am J Surg	2005	31 patients, 50 breasts	2-stage Immediate	Mean age: 42 y	RCS	Standard
Nahabedian,[19] United States	AlloDerm® performance in the setting of prosthetic breast surgery, infection, and irradiation	Plast Reconstr Surg	2009	76 patients, 100 breasts	Mix: revision reconstruction, revision augmentation	Mean age: 46 y	RCS	Standard

(continued on next page)

Table 1
(continued)

Author, Location	Title	Journal	Year	Sample Size	1-Stage vs 2-Stage	Sample Population	Design	Surgical Technique
Namnoum,[20] United States	Expander/implant reconstruction with AlloDerm®: recent experience	*Plast Reconstr Surg*	2009	20 patients, 29 breasts	2-stage Immediate	Mean age: N/D Radiation data not included	RCS	Standard with no SA elevation
Newman et al,[39] United States	The true incidence of near-term postoperative complications in prosthetic breast reconstruction using human ADMs: a meta-analysis	*Aesth Plast Surg*	2011	789 breasts	1-stage 2-stage Immediate	N/D	Meta-analysis	12% overall infection rate on meta-analysis of 12 studies
Parikh,[21] United States	Immediate breast reconstruction with tissue expanders and alloderm	*Plast Reconstr Surg*	2006	43 patients, 58 breasts	2-stage	N/D	RCS	Standard
Premirger et al,[22] United States	The influence of AlloDerm® on expander dynamics and complications in the setting of immediate tissue expander/implant reconstruction: a matched-cohort study	*Ann Plast Surg*	2008	45 patients	2-stage Immediate	Mean age: N/D 6 of 90 patients from both cohorts were radiated preoperatively	RCS matched for TE, RTx, and Dx	Standard with no SA or RA fascia elevation

Study, Country	Title	Journal	Year	Sample	Stage/Timing	Patient/Radiation details	Study type	Comparison
Salzberg,[24] United States	An 8-year experience of direct-to-implant immediate breast reconstruction using human ADM (AlloDerm®)	Plast Reconstr Surg	2011	260 patients, 466 breasts	1-stage Immediate	Mean age: N/D 21 breasts were radiated postoperatively	RCS	Standard
Salzberg,[23] United States	Nonexpansive immediate breast reconstruction using human acellular tissue matrix graft (AlloDerm®)	Ann Plast Surg	2006	49 patients, 76 breasts	1-stage Immediate	Mean age: N/D Radiation data not included	RCS	Standard
Sbitany et al,[25] United States	Acellular dermis-assisted prosthetic breast reconstruction vs complete submuscular coverage: a head-to-head comparison of outcomes	Plast Reconstr Surg	2009	50 patients, 92 breasts	2-stage	Mean age 48 y (SD: 8.6) 6 breasts received postoperative radiation	RCS	Standard
Spear et al,[26] United States	Acellular dermis-assisted breast reconstruction	Aesth Plast Surg	2008	43 patients, 58 breasts	2-stage Immediate	Mean age at stage 1: 50 y (range 36–66 y) 3 breasts were radiated preoperatively 8 breasts were radiated postoperatively	RCS	Standard with no SA, RA, or pectoralis minor elevation

(continued on next page)

Table 1
(continued)

Author, Location	Title	Journal	Year	Sample Size	1-Stage vs 2-Stage	Sample Population	Design	Surgical Technique
Topol et al,[27] Unitec States	Immediate single-stage breast reconstruction using implants and human ADM with adjustment of the lower pole of the breast to reduce unwanted lift	*Ann Plast Surg*	2008	23 patients, 35 breasts	1-stage Immediate	Mean age: N/D Radiation data not included	PCS	Standard with no SA elevation
Uflacke- & Janis,[28] United States	The ADM dermal matrix in the correction of visible parasternal deformities after breast reconstruction	*Plast Reconstr Surg*	2010	1 patient	N/A	Age: 38 y Visible implants in the upper pole	Case report	AlloDerm® used in upper pole to camouflage implant visibility
Zienowicz & Karazaoglu,[29] United States	Implant-based breast reconstruction with allograft	*Plast Reconstr Surg*	2007	24 patients, 30 breasts	1-stage Immediate	Mean age: 47 y (SD: 8) Radiation data not included	PCS	Standard with SA elevation 100% adjustable Spectrum implant

Abbreviations: Dx, diagnosis; N/A, not applicable; N/D, not documented; PCS, prospective case series; RA, rectus abdominis; RCS, retrospective case series; RTx, radiation therapy; SA, serratus anterior; SD, standard deviation; TE, tissue expander.

[a] Standard technique: after the completion of the skin-sparing mastectomies, the inferolateral origin of the pectoralis major muscle is elevated off the anterior chest wall. Using blunt and electrocautery dissection, a subpectoral pocket is developed to the extent of the previously marked perimeter of the breasts. After satisfactory creation of a subpectoral pocket, an appropriately sized piece of ADM is rehydrated in normal saline according to the manufacturer's recommendations. The ADM is sewn along the chest wall at the level of the previously marked inframammary fold and curved laterally and cephalad along the lateral border of the breast perimeter to recreate the natural curvilinear origins of the infero-lateral aspect of the detached pectoralis muscle and breast mound unit.

in breast surgery is AlloDerm®. AlloDerm® is processed via a proprietary deoxycholate/freeze-drying process in which components including types IV and VII collagen, elastin, and laminin are preserved within the residual dermal matrix.[59,60] The ideal ADM lacks immunogenic epitopes and, therefore, evades rejection, absorption, or extrusion.[57] In addition, collagen-dermal scaffolds have the potential to be revascularized, repopulated by fibroblasts, and replaced by autogenous collagen.[60]

Revascularization and Encapsulation

Numerous histologic analyses have shown the potential for human-derived and xenogenic-derived ADM to become incorporated into the host with evidence of revascularization.[60–63] There is also evidence to suggest that some ADMs resist encapsulation, which may be attributable to reduced numbers of myofibroblasts and inflammatory cytokines at the ADM/host interface. It is postulated that the host may not recognize human-derived ADM as foreign, and therefore reacts with a muted inflammatory response.[64–66] This hypothesis may be reflected clinically by reduced capsular contracture rates after ADM-assisted breast surgery. Several series have supported this concept, with low rates of capsular contracture on early follow-up.[7–9,15,20,24,26,27,29]

Postoperative Breast Irradiation

Few clinical studies have examined the use of ADM in the setting of previous or postoperative breast irradiation.[7,12,13,22,24–26] Expanding indications have resulted in increasing numbers of patients who have had breast reconstruction requiring radiotherapy.[67] Multiple investigators have reported higher complication rates, including capsular contracture, infection, and reconstructive failure in tissue expander/implant reconstruction associated with either prereconstruction or postreconstruction radiation.[68–70] Experimental studies have shown favorable results in terms of the ability of ADMs to become vascularized after application to an irradiated bed or after radiation of the ADM itself.[71,72] Komorowska-Timek and colleagues[73] have specifically studied the behavior of ADM around implants in an irradiated, animal model. They found decreased inflammation and pseudoepithelium formation in the presence of an ADM.

Costs of Complications

Differences in capsular contracture rates and outcomes in the setting of irradiation further influence the cost-benefit of use of ADMs in breast surgery. Clinical series examining the effect of radiation in the setting of ADM-assisted breast surgery are scarce and results are conflicting. Antony and colleagues[3] have shown favorable results in the setting of irradiation; however, Spear and colleagues[26] have shown a higher rate of complications. Further basic science and clinical studies are required to evaluate the effects of ADM on capsule formation and behavior in the setting of radiation.

COST CONSIDERATIONS OF ADMs

ADMs come at a significant additional line item cost to the health care system. Introduction of ADMs into practice requires a consideration as to whether the benefits provided are worth spending the limited resources available at a particular institution. This type of evaluation can be conducted from several different viewpoints, such as that of the hospital, the primary payer, or society. The Panel on Cost-Effectiveness in Health and Medicine recommends a societal perspective when conducting cost analyses.[45] This perspective takes into account everyone affected by a particular intervention, whether or not people affected are those who received the intervention.

Proof of Clinical Effectiveness

Before performing an economic analysis, the clinical effectiveness of a new intervention should be proven. Pooling results from multiple randomized controlled trials (RCTs) is the gold standard when evaluating outcomes. Because the number of RCTs comparing surgical interventions is low, surgeons must use data from observational studies with a lower level of evidence and then decide if outcomes from such studies are generalizable to their own practice. In the case of breast surgery, several potential outcomes can be measured, including short-term and long-term complications, aesthetic outcome, patient satisfaction, and patient-reported quality of life. The estimation of costs and effects relies on appropriate measurements. The price of a particular intervention or surgery differs between locations, and thus a particular analyst at 1 institution may reach a different conclusion on cost-effectiveness compared with an analyst in a different country. The estimated cost of a procedure in the United States (multiple third-party payers) is likely not applicable to a surgeon in Canada with 1 surgical fee (1 party payer), which may be a fraction of the equivalent surgical fee in the United States. In addition, when using the societal perspective the cost or charge of a surgical intervention, resource costs such as nursing time and investigations, as well as the cost to other people affected by the intervention must all be taken into account.

Table 2
Use of ADMs in breast aesthetic surgery

Author, Location	Title	Journal	Year	Sample Size	Design	Cost	Technique
Baxter,[30] United States	Intracapsular allogenic dermal grafts for breast implant-related problems	*Plast Reconstr Surg*	2003	10 patients	RCS/Technique paper	N/D	Use of ADM to correct symmastia, bottoming out and rippling in both aesthetic and reconstructive cases
Brown et al,[31] United States	Preventing the "bottoming out" and "star-gazing" phenomena in inferior pedicle breast reduction with an acellular dermal matrix internal brassiere	*Aesth Plast Surg*	2010	27 patients	RCS	N/D	Use of ADM to prevent bottoming out of the breast after Wise-pattern breast reduction
Curtis et al,[32] United States	Use of AlloDerm® for correction of symmastia	*Plast Reconstr Surg*	2010	1 patient	Case report	N/D	Use of medial C-shaped slings of AlloDerm® bilaterally to correct symmastia
Colewell & Breuing,[33] United States	Improving shape and symmetry in mastopexy with autologous or cadaveric dermal slings	*Ann Plast Surg*	2008	10 patients	RCS	N/D	Use of an internal ADM sling to support the breast in mastopexy
Duncan,[34] United States	Correction of implant rippling using allograft dermis	*Aesth Surg J*	2001	34 patients	RCS	N/D	Segmental capsulectomy in the area underlying the rippling to produce a vascularized recipient site for allograft. Allograft was sutured along the inferolateral pectoral muscle edge, placement of implant, and suturing of allograft to the inframammary crease

Hartzell et al,[35] United States	The use of human acellular dermal matrix for the correction of secondary deformities after breast augmentation: results and costs	Plast Reconstr Surg	2010	23 patients, 38 breasts	RCS	Average: $3536–$4856 per breast	Use of human ADM to correct surface irregularities and implant malposition
Maxwell & Gabriel,[36] United States	Use of the acellular dermal matrix in revisionary aesthetic breast surgery	Aesth Surg J	2009	78 patients	RCS	N/D	Use in revision augmentation and revision augmentation mastopexy
Mofid & Singh,[37] United States	Pocket conversion made easy: a simple technique using alloderm to convert subglandular breast implants to the dual-plane position	Aesth Surg J	2009	10 patients, 20 breasts	RCS	N/D	Revision breast augmentation with conversion of subglandular implants to the dual plane position using AlloDerm®
Spear et al,[38] United States	Acellular dermal matrix for the treatment and prevention of implant-associated breast deformities	Plast Reconstr Surg	2011	52 patients, 77 breasts	RCS	N/D	Use of AlloDerm® to correct surface irregularities and implant malposition and to treat capsular contracture

Abbreviations: N/D, not documented; RCS, retrospective case series.

Table 3
ADMs and cost

Name	Manufacturer	Origin	Year Introduced	Shelf Life (y)	Cost per 6-cm × 16-cm-Thick (0.8–1.7 mm) Sheet ($)
AlloDerm®	Lifecell	Human dermal collagen	1994	2	3562
FlexHD®	MTF for Ethicon	Donated acellular human dermis	2005	3	3295
DermaMatrix®	MTF for Synthes CMF	Donated acellular human dermis	2006	3	3295
AlloMax™	Bard Davol	Human dermal collagen	2006	5	4608
SurgiMend®	TEI Biosciences	Fetal bovine dermal collagen	2007	3	Pricing unavailable
Strattice™	Lifecell	Porcine dermal collagen	2008	2	2515[a]

Based on 2011 USD published costs.
DermaMatrix and FlexHD: Mentor 1-800-433-6576.
Abbreviation: MTF, Musculoskeletal Transplant Foundation.
[a] Price of 5-cm × 16-cm sheet as used in breast reconstruction surgery (corresponds to a 6-cm × 16-cm sheet of AlloDerm®).

Formal Cost Evaluation

A formal cost evaluation of the use of ADMs in breast surgery requires knowledge of the cost of the product (**Table 3**), the cost of the surgery being performed, the cost of potential outcomes, costs of patient time expended for the intervention, costs associated with care giving, economic costs borne by employers, and costs borne by the rest of society, also known as friction costs, associated with absenteeism.[44] In addition, it is essential to determine the probabilities of all relevant outcomes and whether outcomes with the use of ADMs differ from outcomes with the alternative techniques. With only 27 published series on the use of ADMs in breast reconstructive surgery and 9 published series in breast aesthetic surgery, it is difficult to know with certainty if outcomes using ADMs are better, worse, or equivalent to outcomes without the use of ADMs. Formal RCTs evaluating surgery with and without ADMs are required to make this determination. A summary of current published outcomes with use of ADMs in both reconstructive and aesthetic breast surgery follows.

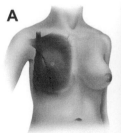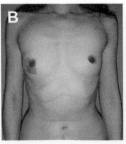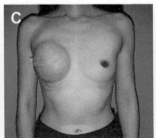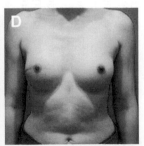

Fig. 2. Traditional 2-stage alloplastic breast reconstruction. (*A*) Total submuscular coverage of a tissue expander with pectoralis major medially and pectoralis minor/serratus anterior sling laterally. (*B*) 45-year-old patient who underwent right total submuscular 2-stage reconstruction without ADM. (*C*) Tissue expander phase shows high-riding tissue expander, tight inferolateral pocket, and lack of projection. (*D*) Postoperative result shown after extensive capsulotomies at second stage (style 15: 339 g Allergan implant) and left breast augmentation (style 10: 180 g Allergan implant).

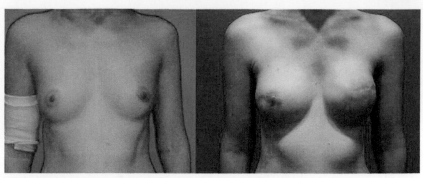

Fig. 3. One-stage and 2-stage alloplastic breast reconstruction using ADM. 38-year-old patient who underwent nipple-areola complex-sparing stage reconstruction using AlloDerm® (6 × 16 cm) on the right (style 15: 265-g Allergan implant) and 2-stage reconstruction using AlloDerm® (6 × 16 cm) on the left. Photograph is after radiation and implant exchange on the left (style 20: 325-g Allergan implant).

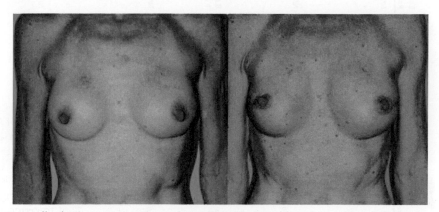

Fig. 4. One-stage alloplastic reconstruction using ADM. 53-year-old patient with existing subpectoral saline implants, diagnosed with left ductal carcinoma in situ, and underwent bilateral nipple-areola complex-sparing mastectomies with 1-stage reconstruction using AlloDerm® (6 × 16 cm) and cohesive gel implants (FX120: 360 g Allergan implant).

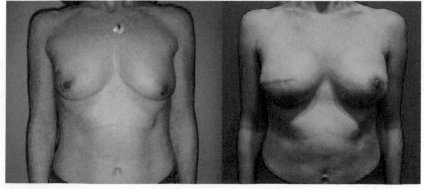

Fig. 5. One-stage and 2-stage alloplastic breast reconstruction using ADM. 41-year-old patient who underwent nipple-areola complex-sparing 1-stage reconstruction using AlloDerm® (6 × 16 cm) on the left (style MF: 335 g Allergan implant) and 2-stage reconstruction using AlloDerm® (6 × 16 cm) on the right (style MF: 335 g Allergan implant).

Table 4
Outcomes in breast reconstruction surgery using ADMs

Author, Location	Title	ADM	Sample Size	Follow-up	Mastectomy Flap Necrosis and Revision	Capsular Contracture	Late Revision Rate	Seroma Rate	Infection Rate	Implant Extrusion or Autologous Salvage
Antony et al,[3] United States	ADM implantation in 153 immediate two-stage tissue expander breast reconstructions: determining the incidence and significant predictors of complications	AlloDerm® 4 × 16 cm	96 patients, 153 breasts	N/D	4.6%	N/D	N/D	7.2%	3.3%	5.9%
Ashikari et al,[4] United States	Subcutaneous mastectomy and immediate reconstruction for prevention of breast cancer for high-risk patients	AlloDerm® 4 × 12 cm	65 patients, 130 breasts 1-stage	4.6 y (SD: 56 mo)	N/D	N/D	N/D	N/D	0%	N/D
Austen et al,[5] United States	A simplified technique for single stage breast reconstruction	AlloDerm® 4 × 12 cm 4 × 16 cm	25 patients, 35 breasts 1-stage	10 mo	5.7% 2 cases revised in office setting	N/D	8.6% 1 implant exchanged for asymmetry, 1 for rippling	N/D	N/D	2.9%
Becker et al,[6] United States	AlloDerm® vs DermaMatrix® in immediate expander-based breast reconstruction: a preliminary comparison of complication profiles and material compliance	AlloDerm® 25 breasts DermaMatrix® 25 breasts	30 patients, 50 breasts 2-stage	6.7 mo	0%	N/D	N/D	4% 1 breast in DermaMatrix® group	4% 1 breast in DermaMatrix® group	0%
Bindingnavele et al[7] United States	Use of ADM and tissue expansion in postmastectomy breast reconstruction	AlloDerm®	41 patients, 65 breasts 2-stage	10 mo (range: 7–21 mo)	0%	0%	N/D	4.6%	3.1%	1.5%
Breuing et al,[8] United States	Immediate bilateral breast reconstruction with implants and inferolateral AlloDerm® slings	AlloDerm® 4–6 × 14–16 cm	10 patients, 20 breasts 1-stage	6 mo–1 y	5% Revised in office setting	0%	0%	0%	0%	0%

Study	Title	ADM	Patients	Follow-up						
Breuing and Colwell,[9] United States	Inferolateral AlloDerm® hammock for implant coverage in breast reconstruction	AlloDerm®	43 patients, 67 breasts 1-stage 2-stage Delayed Revisional	6 m–3 y	N/D	0%	N/D	0%	3%	1.5%
Chen et al,[10] United States	A novel cost-saving approach to the use of ADM (AlloDerm®) in postmastectomy breast and nipple reconstructions	AlloDerm® 6 × 16 cm	13 patients, 23 breasts 2-stage	N/D	N/D	N/D	N/D	N/D	N/D	N/D
Chun et al,[11] United States	Implant-based breast reconstruction using ADM and the risk of postoperative complications	AlloDerm®	269 breasts 1-stage 2-stage	N/D	23.4%	N/D	N/D	14.1%	8.9%	5.9%
Derderian et al,[12] United States	Wise-pattern breast reconstruction modification using alloderm and a vascularized dermal-subcutaneous pedicle	AlloDerm®	20 patients 2-stage	N/D	25% wound breakdown at T junction All treated nonoperatively	N/D	0%	N/D	N/D	0%
Gamboa-Bobadilla,[14] United States	Implant breast reconstruction using ADM	AlloDerm® 4 × 16 cm	11 patients, 13 breasts 1-stage	14 mo	N/D	N/D	N/D	7.7%	7.7%	7.7%
Lanier et al,[15] United States	The effect of ADM use on complication rates in tissue expander/implant breast reconstruction	AlloDerm® Strattice™ FlexHD® 6 × 16 cm 8 × 16 cm	52 breasts 2-stage	6.8 mo (SD: 2.8 mo)	15.4%	3.9%	25%	15.4%	28.9%	19.2%
Liu et al,[16] United States	Postoperative complications in prosthesis-based breast reconstruction using ADM	AlloDerm®	192 patients, 266 breasts 2-stage	N/D	13.9%	N/D	N/D	7.1%	6.8%	4.9%
Losken,[17] United States	Early results using sterilized ADM (neoform) in post-mastectomy tissue expander breast reconstruction	Surgimend (previously Neoform™) 4 × 16 6 × 16	22 patients, 31 breasts 2-stage	10.2 mo (range: 6-16 mo)	3.2% Managed in office setting	N/D	N/D	0%	0%	0%
Margulies et al,[18] United States	Total skin-sparing mastectomy without preservation of the nipple-areola complex	AlloDerm®	31 patients, 50 breasts 2-stage	7.9 mo (SD: 5.4 mo)	14%	N/D	N/D	N/D	4%	N/D

(continued on next page)

Table 4
(continued)

Author, Location	Title	ADM	Sample Size	Follow-up	Mastectomy Flap Necrosis and Revision	Capsular Contracture	Late Revision Rate	Seroma Rate	Infection Rate	Implant Extrusion or Autologous Salvage
Nahabedian et al,[19] United States	AlloDerm® performance in the setting of prosthetic breast surgery, infection, and irradiation	AlloDerm®	76 patients, 100 breasts 2-stage	17 mo (range: 6–37 mo)	3%	N/D	N/D	5%	5%	2%
Namnoum,[20] United States	Expander/implant reconstruction with AlloDerm®: recent experience	AlloDerm® 4 × 16 cm 4 × 12 cm	20 patients, 29 breasts 2-stage	21 mo (range: 3–32 mo)	3.4%	0%	0%	3.4%	3.4%	0%
Parikh,[21] United States	Immediate breast reconstruction with tissue expanders and AlloDerm®	AlloDerm®	43 patients, 58 breasts	N/D	5.2%	N/D	N/D	3.4%	5.2%	1.7%
Preminger et al,[22] United States	The influence of AlloDerm® on expander dynamics and complications in the setting of immediate tissue expander/implant reconstruction: a matched-cohort study	AlloDerm®	45 breasts 2-stage	N/D	N/D	N/D	N/D	6.7%	2.2%	0%
Salzberg,[24] United States	An 8-year experience of direct-to-implant immediate breast reconstruction using human ADM (AlloDerm®)	AlloDerm®	260 patients, 466 breasts 1-stage	28.9 mo (SD: 21.3 mo)	1.1%	0.4% Both cases (2) required operative intervention	9.4% Most frequent revision was to increase implant size	N/D	0.2%	1.3%
Salzberg,[23] United States	Nonexpansive immediate breast reconstruction using ADM (AlloDerm®)	AlloDerm®	49 patients, 76 breasts 1-stage	18 months (Range: 3–52 months)	3.9% Two nonoperatively, 1 managed operatively	0%	N/D	0%	0%	0%
Sbitany et al,[25] United States	ADM-assisted prosthetic breast reconstruction vs complete submuscular coverage: a head-to-head comparison of outcomes	AlloDerm®	50 patientss 92 breasts 2-stage	N/D	N/D	N/D	N/D	6%	8%	8%

Study	Description	Material	Follow-up						
Spear et al,[26] United States	ADM-assisted breast reconstruction	AlloDerm® 4 × 12 cm 4 × 16 cm	25.9 mo (range: 19.2–35.3 mo)	3.4%	2%	1.7%	4%	6.9%	12.1% (Conversion to autologous salvage at second stage without implant extrusion)
Topol et al,[27] United States	Immediate single-stage breast reconstruction using implants and ADM with adjustment of the lower pole of the breast to reduce unwanted lift	AlloDerm® 4 × 16 cm	9.5 mo (range: 1–24 mo)	0%	0%	0%	N/D	8.6%	5.7%
Zienowicz and Karacaoglu,[29] United States	Implant-based breast reconstruction with allograft	AlloDerm®	18 mo (range: 15–24 mo)	20% All managed nonoperatively	0%	0%	0%	0%	0%
Overall weighted average by breast (mix)[a]	—	—	—	8.1% 148/1818	0.5% 5/898	6.5% 96/1484	9% 62/710	4.3% 92/2130	3.5% 69/1985
Overall weighted average by breast (1-stage)[b]	—	—	—	2.6% 17/662	0.3% 2/627	0.5% 1/174	8.5% 47/551	0.6% 5/770	1.5% 10/675
Overall weighted average by breast (2-stage)[b]	—	—	—	7.9% 74/932	1.4% 3/204	5.8% 58/999	9.4% 15/159	5.8% 61/1049	4.6% 47/1019
Allergan core study for primary reconstruction (7-y follow-up)[47] N = 98 patients	—	—	—	2.3%	17.1%	N/D	53.3%	3.2%	7.7%
Mentor core study for primary reconstruction (3-y follow-up)[48] N = 251 patients	—	—	—	N/D	8.3%	4.9%	27%	5.7%	5.7%

Note: weighted averages calculated by breast.

Abbreviations: ADM, acellular dermal matrix; N/D, not documented; SD, standard deviation.

[a] Studies with one and two-stage reconstruction or a mix of one- and two-stage reconstruction.

[b] Studies with a mix of one and two-stage reconstructions not included in weighted average.

SUMMARY OF OUTCOMES OF USE OF ADMs IN RECONSTRUCTIVE BREAST SURGERY

Traditionally, 2-stage immediate alloplastic breast reconstruction has involved total submuscular coverage of a tissue expander to prevent implant exposure, improve implant coverage, and to allow for control of the inframammary fold (**Fig. 2**A). Problems with this technique include high-riding tissue expanders, loss of expansion of the infero-lateral pocket secondary to tightness of the serratus anterior, and limited breast projection. Satisfactory results may be achieved with aggressive capsulotomies at the time of implant exchange (see **Fig. 2**D). Attempts to eliminate the problems seen with traditional total submuscular coverage have led to the incorporation of ADMs into 2-stage alloplastic reconstructions, and in the appropriate patient, incorporation of ADM may allow for elimination of the tissue-expansion phase completely (1-stage reconstruction, **Figs. 3–5**).

Clinical Outcomes

Before assessing the cost-benefit of these techniques compared with the traditional approach, the probabilities of clinically important outcomes must be assessed. One must then determine whether outcomes with the use of ADMs compare favorably with those seen with the traditional approach. There have been 25 published series (case reports excluded) that include data on both 1-stage and 2-stage alloplastic breast reconstruction using ADMs.[3,5–12,14–27,29] **Table 4** summarizes the rates of mastectomy flap necrosis, late revision, capsular contracture, seroma, infection, and implant loss for these series. We have calculated the weighted average for each of these outcomes by breast (for patients with 1-stage and 2-stage reconstructions combined, 1-stage reconstruction only, and 2-stage reconstruction only) and compared these outcomes with those with traditional 2-stage reconstruction reported in the Allergan[74] and Mentor[75] core studies. On short-term follow-up, addition of ADMs to alloplastic breast reconstruction (1-stage and 2-stage reconstruction using ADM outcomes combined) seems to result in favorable outcomes for capsular contracture, late revision, and total implant loss compared with traditional 2-stage (non-ADM) reconstruction. Rates of mastectomy flap necrosis, seroma, and infection are slightly higher than those seen in the core studies.

1-Stage (with ADM) and 2-Stage (non-ADM) Reconstruction Weighted Averages

We also calculated the weighted averages for 1-stage (with ADM) versus 2-stage reconstruction without ADM (see **Table 4**). This calculation reveals lower rates of:

- capsular contracture
- late revision
- seroma
- infection
- implant loss

and similar rates of mastectomy flap necrosis for 1-stage reconstruction with ADMs when compared with the traditional technique reported in the core studies.

Two-stage reconstruction using ADMs seems to confer a lower rate of:

- capsular contracture
- revision and implant loss

but higher rates of:

- mastectomy flap necrosis
- seroma
- infection

when compared with the core study results (see **Table 4**).

Overall, limited case series and insufficient follow-up times have been reported in the literature. Definitive comparisons therefore cannot be made. However, based on these studies, use of ADMs in alloplastic breast reconstruction seems to be a safe alternative, with some possible benefits compared with the traditional, non-ADM approach.

Cost Considerations

Assuming that results are comparable with the traditional 2-stage alloplastic approach, one must then consider cost. Most published series have used a 6-cm × 16-cm sheet of AlloDerm®, which is priced at $3562 (US dollars, 2011 pricing, LifeCell Corporation, Branchburg, NJ, USA). Addition of this ADM to a 2-stage reconstruction increases the overall cost of a unilateral procedure by this amount. Whether this cost is offset by reduction in costs of subsequent procedures (possible lower rates of late revision, capsular contracture, and implant loss/conversion to autologous reconstruction) needs to be assessed in a formal cost analysis ideally using outcomes generated from an RCT comparing the 2 techniques. Follow-up for procedures using ADMs is too short to be reliably compared with the 7-year follow-up for traditional 2-stage reconstruction of the Allergan core study. In addition, the patients included in the weighted averages for outcomes by breast included in **Table 4** come from a diverse number of institutions and therefore surgical procedures vary and weighted averages serve only as an estimate for outcomes data. Combining heterogeneous samples to make definitive large-scale conclusions is not reliable. Therefore, the outcomes listed in **Table 4** can only be used as a guide from the current published literature.

Comparison of Traditional 2-Stage Reconstruction with Alloplastic 1-Stage Reconstruction

Conversion of traditional 2-stage total submuscular alloplastic reconstruction to 1-stage alloplastic reconstruction using ADMs results in cost savings. This situation results from elimination of the cost of the tissue expander and second-stage surgery. In a recent Canadian cost analysis, the cost of a 1-stage implant reconstruction with no complications was estimated at $10,239.85 and that of a noncomplicated 2-stage non-ADM reconstruction at $10,584.05.[41] If outcomes are better with the 1-stage approach, further cost savings may be anticipated.

The cost tool published by Jansen and Macadam in 2011[41] allows for an estimation of costs of 1-stage reconstruction using ADM versus traditional 2-stage reconstruction without ADM in a Canadian health care setting (available for download with article). The ADM used in this model was a 6-cm × 16-cm sheet of AlloDerm®. Inputting the weighted averages of outcomes for 1-stage

reconstruction using ADM listed in **Table 4** and the average of outcomes listed by the Allergan core study (rate for implant exposure with salvage estimated and rate for seroma in 2-stage reconstruction inputted from Mentor core study), the cost of 1-stage reconstruction including complications becomes $11,115 and that of traditional 2-stage reconstruction including complications becomes $15,054 (**Fig. 6**).

Another recent cost analysis published from an American institution estimated the cost of traditional 2-stage reconstruction at $10,934 and that of 1-stage reconstruction with ADM at $5423. Notable differences of this cost analysis when compared with the Canadian study were the inputted cost of ADM at just $321 (Medicare fee) and significant differences in hospital fees and surgical fees between 2-stage and 1-stage reconstruction. Jansen and Macadam estimated equivalent hospital fees for each technique (both requiring 1 night in hospital), whereas de Blacam and colleagues estimated a $3000 difference in hospital fees. De Blacam and colleagues estimated a $2000 difference in surgical fees between the 2 techniques, whereas Jansen and Macadam estimated a $500 difference. This observation highlights the differences in costs across different institutions.

Using the limited outcomes data available, it seems that conversion to 1-stage reconstruction, in the appropriate patient, may result in a cost benefit according to these cost-minimization approaches.

Hourly OR cost ($)	$ 2,100
Cost for one day in hospital ($)	$ 1,200
TE Cost ($)	$ 1,400
Implant material cost ($)	$ 900
AlloDerm material cost ($)	$ 3,651

Procedure	Expected Cost	Baseline Cost
Direct-to-implant with AD	$ 11,115	$ 10,240
Two stage without AD	$ 15,054	$ 10,584

Procedures	OR Time (Hrs)	Stay in Hospital (Days)	Procedure Billing Code ($)	Material Cost	Total Cost
TE Reconstruction (no AD)	2	1	$495.20	$ 1,400	$ 7,295.20
Implant Exchange	1	0	$288.85	$ 900	$ 3,288.85
Implant + AD 1-Stage Reconstruction	2	1	$288.85	$ 4,551	$ 10,239.85
Exposure with Loss - Implant removal, I&D	1	0	$441.83	$	$ 2,541.83
Exposure with Loss - Latiss TE Reconstruction	4.5	2	$1,241.68	$ 1,400	$ 14,491.68
Exposure with Loss - Implant Exchange	1	0	$288.85	$ 900	$ 3,288.85
Exposure with Salvage	1	0	$128.44	$ -	$ 2,228.44
Hematoma	1	1	$118.15	$ -	$ 3,418.15
Seroma	0	0	$0.00	$ -	$ -
Marginal flap necrosis	0	0	$0.00	$ 50	$ 50.00
Capsular Constracture	1	0	$339.15	$ 900	$ 3,339.15
Revisions	1.5	0	$288.85	$ 900	$ 4,338.85

Outcomes and Probabilities	Direct-to-implant AD	Two Stage non AD
Implant exposure with loss	1.5%	7.7%
Implant exposure with salvage	4.0%	4.0%
Infection	0.6%	3.2%
Hematoma	3.0%	2.0%
Seroma	0.5%	4.9%
Marginal flap necrosis	2.6%	2.3%
Capsular Contracture	0.3%	17.1%
Revisions	8.5%	53.3%

AD=AlloDerm
OR=operating room
TE=tissue expander

Fig. 6. One-stage AlloDerm® reconstruction and two-stage non-alloDerm® reconstruction calculator. Upper right box with costs in green show expected costs for one-stage (direct-to-implant) versus traditional two-stage reconstruction after inputting weighted averages for outcomes from **Table 4** and core study outcomes for the two-stage non-ADM group. Outcome probability for exposure with salvage is estimated at 4% for both groups. Hematoma probability estimated at 3% for one-stage reconstruction.

Table 5
Early experience with 1-stage reconstruction using ACD at the University of British Columbia

Author, Location	ADM	Sample Size	Follow-up	Mastectomy Flap Necrosis Requiring Revision	Capsular Contracture	Late Revision Rate	Seroma Rate	Infection Rate	Implant Extrusion or Autologous Salvage
Macadam & Lennox,[a] Canada	AlloDerm® 6 × 16 cm	34 patients, 51 breasts 1-stage Nonradiated	3–18 mo	19%	7.7% 4 breasts all requiring surgical intervention	23% 4 breasts for capsular contracture, 2 breasts for rippling (conversion to cohesive gel), 2 breasts for chronic pain leading to removal of implants, 4 breasts for implant malposition or size	3.8%	0%	5.8% 3 cases secondary to mastectomy flap necrosis. Two managed with latissimus flap, 1 with deep inferior epigastric perforator flap
Overall weighted average from **Table 4** by breast (1-stage)	—	—	—	2.6% 17/662	0.3% 2/627	8.5% 47/551	0.5% 1/174	0.6% 5/770	1.5% 10/675
Allergan core study for primary reconstruction[47] (7-y follow-up)	—	—	—	2.3%	17.1%	53.3%	N/D	3.2%	7.7%
Mentor core study for primary reconstruction[48] (3-y follow-up)	—	—	—	N/D	8.3%	27%	4.9%	5.7%	5.7%

Abbreviation: N/D, not documented.
Patients who received radiation excluded.
[a] Macadam SA and Lennox PA, unpublished data, 2010–2011.

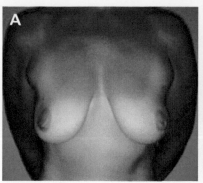
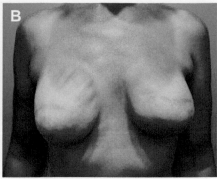

Fig. 7. One-stage reconstruction using ADM with implant displacement. 46 year-old patient (*A*) who underwent bilateral 1-stage reconstruction using AlloDerm® (6 × 16 cm) and cohesive gel implants (MX: 410 g Allergan implant). Postoperative photo shown (*B*) after radiation on the left and implant displacement with surface irregularities on the right.

Further studies with longer-term follow-up are required to examine this issue more rigorously.

Other Considerations in Cost Analysis of Alloplastic Reconstruction

One caveat of this type of analysis is the significant learning curve that may be associated with introduction of single-stage breast reconstruction into practice. Choice of the appropriate patient may affect early complication rates, and therefore surgeons may experience higher complication rates within the early phase of performing 1-stage surgery. We list our 12-month complication profile for consecutive nonirradiated patients undergoing 1-stage reconstruction using AlloDerm® in **Table 5**. Within this first 12-month period, we noted a high rate of mastectomy flap necrosis (19%), which led to 3 cases of implant extrusion and conversion to an autologous procedure (5.8%). In addition, our revision rate of 23% reflects difficulty with initial implant selection, a 7.7% rate of early grade 3/4 capsular contracture, and 4 cases of implant malposition/size change (**Fig. 7**). Higher overall complications in the early learning curve period may inflate the cost of 1-stage surgery using ADMs initially.

REVISIONARY AESTHETIC BREAST SURGERY

Revisionary aesthetic breast surgery is complex and unpredictable. The Allergan core study reports a 41% revision rate after a first revisionary surgery after breast augmentation.[74] Revisions result in increased cost to the patient and potentially to the surgeon. Surgeons must address several different issues, including thinning of tissues secondary to placement of large prostheses, surface irregularities, symmastia, implant displacement, and most commonly capsular contracture. Traditionally, techniques such as creation of a neopocket to facilitate site change, capsulorrhaphy, use of capsular flaps, fat grafting, and conversion to form-stable prostheses have been used with varying degrees of success in revisional aesthetic breast surgery.[76–81] Use of ADMs in aesthetic breast surgery has become common in recent years. Reported uses include creation of a medial barrier to implant migration in symmastia correction, provision of coverage and support in the lower pole when performing a neosubpectoral dual plane site change, incorporation into the upper pole to camouflage surface irregularities, and provision of an interface when performing

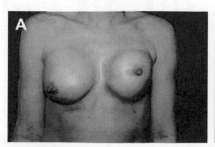
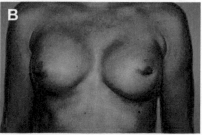

Fig. 8. 41-year-old patient (*A*) who underwent multiple surgeries on the left breast for recurrent capsular contracture after augmentation with subpectoral saline implants. She underwent revision with total capsulectomy and AlloDerm® as a sling in the lower pole. Postoperative photograph (*B*) taken at 5-month follow-up.

Table 6
Outcomes in breast aesthetic surgery using ADMs

Author, Location	Title	ADM	Sample Size	Follow-up	Capsular Contracture	Revision Rate	Seroma Rate	Infection Rate	Total Loss
Baxter,[30] United States	Intracapsular allogenic dermal grafts for breast implant-related problems	AlloDerm®	10 patients	6–24 mo	0%	20% One case of bottoming out, and 1 case with relapse of symmastia	0%	0%	0%
Brown et al,[31] United States	Preventing the "bottoming out" and "star-gazing" phenomena in inferior pedicle breast reduction with an ADM internal brassiere	AlloDerm®	27 patients 54 breasts	19 mo (range: 5–29 mo)	N/A	0%	N/D	3.7%	N/A
Colewell & Breuing,[33] United States	Improving shape and symmetry in mastopexy with ADM slings	Autologous dermal grafts in 5 patients AlloDerm® in 5 patients 4 × 16 cm	10 patients	6 mo–3 y	N/A	0%	0%	0%	N/A
Duncan,[34] United States	Correction of implant rippling using allograft dermis	AlloDerm® Dermaplant 4 × 12 cm 4 × 8 cm	34 patients	18 mo	2.9%	5.9%	0%	2.9%	0%
Hartzell et al,[35] United States	The use of human ADM for the correction of secondary deformities after breast augmentation: results and costs	AlloDerm® 1.13 sheets per patient $3536 to $4856 per breast per operation	23 patients 38 breasts	25 mo (range: 4–66 mo)	0% recurrence	15.8% For persistent surface irregularities in 2 patients (4 breasts received additional ADM) and larger implants in 1 patient	0%	2.6%	0%

Study	Description	Patients/breasts	ADM	Follow-up						
Maxwell & Gabriel,[36] United States	Use of the ADM in revisionary aesthetic breast surgery	78 patients 156 breasts	AlloDerm® Strattice™ FlexHD® DermaMatrix® SurgiMend®	12 mo	0%	0.64%	0%	1.3%	0%	0%
Mofid & Singh,[37] United States	Pocket conversion made easy: a simple technique using alloderm to convert subglandular breast implants to the dual-plane position	10 patients 20 breasts	AlloDerm® 4 × 16 cm	12 mo	N/D	0%	N/D	N/D	N/D	N/D
Spear et al,[38] United States	ADM for the treatment and prevention of implant-associated breast deformities	52 patients 77 breasts	AlloDerm® Strattice™	8.6 mo	N/D	4%	1.3%	1.3%	5.2%	1.3%
Weighted average by breast	—	—	—	—	0.4% 1/228	3.3% 10/301	1% 3/281	0.4% 1/271	2% 5/271	0.4% 1/271
Allergan core study complication rates for revision augmentation (7-y follow-up)[47] N = 147 patients	—	—	—	—		20.4%	40.5%	6.1%	1.4%	4.3%
Mentor core study for revision augmentation (3-y follow-up)[48] N = 146 patients	—	—	—	—		18.9%	28%	2.1%	1.4%	5.9%

Abbreviations: N/A, not applicable; N/D, not documented.

capsulotomies for recurrent capsular contracture (**Fig. 8**). It has been postulated that incorporation of ADMs into the breast pocket may result in a lower rate of capsular contracture.[66,73]

Patients undergoing aesthetic breast surgery have high expectations, and cost is a significant concern. It is therefore incumbent on the surgeon to provide revisionary surgery that has a high probability of success. As with reconstructive breast surgery using ADMs, aesthetic breast surgery case series reporting on the use of ADMs are rare. There are only 9 case series in the literature, with a maximum follow-up of 25 months. **Table 6** summarizes the probabilities of capsular contracture, revision, seroma, infection, and implant loss for these studies. These series are heterogeneous and therefore weighted averages serve only as a rough estimate to guide comparisons; however, comparison with outcomes of the Allergan and Mentor core studies show a lower rate of all complications except infection when using ADMs at the first revision surgery.

This situation has the most impact when one considers revision and capsular contracture. The Allergan core study reports a 40.5% revision rate and a 20.4% capsular contracture rate after revision of augmentation at 7 years. This finding is compared with the 0.4% (capsular contracture) and 3.3% (revision) weighted average rates seen in **Table 6**. If use of ADMs at the initial revision surgery saves the patient additional revisionary surgeries, the cost of the ADMs is offset. This potential cost saving needs to be examined more rigorously, with larger, homogeneous series with longer follow-up.

AUTHOR'S INSTITUTIONAL EXPERIENCE

At our institution, introduction of ADMs into breast surgery practice required a detailed proposal including a literature review and preliminary cost analysis. The cost savings that would be achieved with conversion to 1-stage reconstruction with ADM in appropriate patients was highlighted. In our experience, approximately 30% to 40% of alloplastic breast reconstruction candidates are appropriate for 1-stage reconstruction using ADM (small to medium breast size, mild to moderate ptosis, good skin elasticity). Within our breast surgery program, this percentage translates to 50 alloplastic breast reconstruction patients per year. Assuming comparable or lower complication rates with the use of ADM, this situation would create cost savings for our institution by eliminating the cost of the second-stage surgery, the cost of the tissue expander device, and potentially further revisional surgery.

We performed a systematic review to determine probabilities for clinically relevant outcomes after alloplastic breast reconstruction. A decision analytical model was used to estimate the cost for 1-stage reconstruction with AlloDerm® versus traditional 2-stage reconstruction.[41] This is a formal quantitative method used to assess the relative

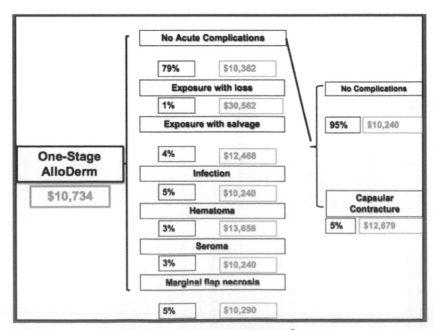

Fig. 9. Decision tree for cost of 1-stage reconstruction with AlloDerm®.

value of uncertain clinical outcomes. A decision tree with various potential clinical outcomes and assigned probabilities based on the systematic review was created (**Fig. 9**). In the case shown in **Fig. 9**, the implied probability of no acute complications is 79% and late capsular contracture rate is 5%. Working backward, expected cost as a probability-weighted average is calculated. For 1-stage reconstruction, the expected cost with the original estimated complication probabilities is $10,734. In the same model, the cost of 2-stage reconstruction was $11,251. Sensitivity analyses showed that with an ADM cost less than $4168 and a 1-stage surgery of duration less than 2.25 hours, 1-stage reconstruction was less costly than 2-stage reconstruction. Use of the weighted averages from outcomes shown in **Table 4** produces an even greater cost saving ($11,074 vs $15,054). Sensitivity analyses using these outcomes have not been performed. These costs are based on a Canadian health care single-payer system and therefore cannot be extrapolated to US institutions.

Based on this initial analysis, preliminary approval for use of ADMs in breast reconstructive surgery was obtained at our institution. Clinical data are compiled in a database prospectively so that outcomes can be monitored and interim cost analyses performed.

SUMMARY OF USE OF ADMs IN BREAST SURGERY

The use of ADMs in reconstructive and aesthetic breast surgery should be compared with standard alternatives using a formal cost-effectiveness analysis. This analysis offers more complete information about the size and value of health effects and costs. However, no method of health care decision making captures all issues such as medical necessity, standards of evidence, fairness, and expected benefit.

Clinical equipoise exists with respect to the use of ADMs in breast surgery. Limited case series cannot definitively show a benefit, and therefore the surgeon is left to decide if ADMs should be incorporated into practice, with little guidance from the literature. Two RCTs are under way (McCarthy and colleagues at Memorial Sloan Kettering Cancer Center comparing 2-stage breast reconstruction with and without ADM; and Zhong and colleagues at the University of Toronto comparing 1-stage breast reconstruction with ADM with 2-stage breast reconstruction without ADM). When evaluating 1-stage reconstruction with ADM versus 2-stage reconstruction without ADM, outcomes need to be compared between patients who would be candidates for both 1-

stage and 2-stage reconstruction because these women generally have a low body mass index (calculated as weight in kilograms divided by the square of height in meters) and smaller breasts, and therefore may be at lower risk for complications than patients who would only be candidates for 2-stage reconstruction. The results of these RCTs will provide outcomes data that can then be applied to a formal cost analysis. In addition, in the future, patient-reported outcomes data may facilitate a cost-utility analysis. This analysis provides definitive information that decision makers can use as an aid in weighing the relative benefits of use of ADMs in breast surgery. A similar scenario for aesthetic breast surgery is less likely because private-pay patients are generally unwilling to enter into an RCT. In this setting, large prospective observational studies with standardized techniques are required to evaluate outcomes over the long-term to determine the impact of ADMs on costs of aesthetic breast surgery.

REFERENCES

1. Birnbaum L. Use of dermal grafts to cover implants in breast reconstructions. Plast Reconstr Surg 1979; 63(4):487–91.
2. Maguina P, Hoffman R, Szczerba S. Autologous dermal graft in breast reconstruction and treatment of breast implant malposition. Plast Reconstr Surg 2010;125(4):170e–1e.
3. Antony AK, McCarthy CM, Cordeiro PG, et al. Acellular human dermis implantation in 153 immediate two-stage tissue expander breast reconstructions: determining the incidence and significant predictors of complications. Plast Reconstr Surg 2010;125: 1606–14.
4. Ashikari RH, Ashikari AY, Kelemen PR, et al. Subcutaneous mastectomy and immediate reconstruction for prevention of breast cancer for high-risk patients. Breast Cancer 2008;15:185–91.
5. Austen WG, Hartzell TL, Hertl MC. A simplified technique for single stage breast reconstruction. Poster presented at: 2006 New England Surgical Society Meeting. Groton, September 16, 2006.
6. Becker S, Saint-Cyr M, Wong C, et al. AlloDerm versus DermaMatrix in immediate expander-based breast reconstruction: a preliminary comparison of complication profiles and material compliance. Plast Reconstr Surg 2009;123:1–6 [discussion: 107–8].
7. Bindingnavele V, Gaon M, Ota KS, et al. Use of acellular cadaveric dermis and tissue expansion in postmastectomy breast reconstruction. J Plast Reconstr Aesthet Surg 2007;60:1214–8.
8. Breuing KH, Warren SM. Immediate bilateral breast reconstruction with implants and inferolateral AlloDerm slings. Ann Plast Surg 2005;55:232–9.

9. Breuing KH, Colwell AS. Inferolateral AlloDerm hammock for implant coverage in breast reconstruction. Ann Plast Surg 2007;59:250–5.

10. Chen WF, Barounis D, Kalimuthu R. A novel cost-saving approach to the use of acellular dermal matrix (AlloDerm) in postmastectomy breast and nipple reconstructions. Plast Reconstr Surg 2010; 125(2):479–81.

11. Chun YS, Verma K, Rosen H, et al. Implant-based breast reconstruction using acellular dermal matrix and the risk of postoperative complications. Plast Reconstr Surg 2010;125(2):429–36.

12. Derderian CA, Karp NS, Choi M. Wise-pattern breast reconstruction: modification using AlloDerm and a vascularized dermal-subcutaneous pedicle. Ann Plast Surg 2009;62:528–32.

13. Ellsworth WA, Rizvi M, Lypka M, et al. Breast implant salvage with the use of acellular dermal matrix following partial mastectomy. Plast Reconstr Surg 2010;126(4):189e–90e.

14. Gamboa-Bobadilla GM. Implant breast reconstruction using acellular dermal matrix. Ann Plast Surg 2006;56(1):22–5.

15. Lanier ST, Wang ED, Chen JJ, et al. The effect of acellular dermal matrix use on complication rates in tissue expander/implant breast reconstruction. Ann Plast Surg 2010;64(5):674–8.

16. Liu AS, Kao HK, Reish RG, et al. Postoperative complications in prosthesis-based breast reconstruction using acellular dermal matrix. Plast Reconstr Surg 2011;127(5):1755–62.

17. Losken A. Early results using sterilized acellular human dermis (NeoForm) in postmastectomy tissue expander breast reconstruction. Plast Reconstr Surg 2006;123(6):1654–8.

18. Margulies AG, Hochberg J, Kepple J, et al. Total skin-sparing mastectomy without preservation of the nipple-areola complex. Am J Surg 2005;190:907–12.

19. Nahabedian MY. AlloDerm performance in the setting of prosthetic breast surgery, infection, and irradiation. Plast Reconstr Surg 2009;124(6):1743–53.

20. Namnoum JD. Expander/implant reconstruction with AlloDerm: recent experience. Plast Reconstr Surg 2009;124(2):387–94.

21. Parikh PM, Spear SL, Menon N, et al. Immediate breast reconstruction with tissue expanders and alloderm. Plast Reconstr Surg 2006;118(Suppl 4):18.

22. Preminger BA, McCarthy CM, Hu QY, et al. The influence of AlloDerm on expander dynamics and complications in the setting of immediate tissue expander/implant reconstruction: a matched-cohort study. Ann Plast Surg 2008;60:510–3.

23. Salzberg CA. Nonexpansive immediate breast reconstruction using human acellular tissue matrix graft (AlloDerm). Ann Plast Surg 2006;57:1–5.

24. Salzberg CA, Ashikari AY, Koch RM, et al. An 8-year experience of direct-to-implant immediate breast reconstruction using human acellular dermal matrix (AlloDerm). Plast Reconstr Surg 2011;127(2): 514–24.

25. Sbitany H, Sandeen SN, AMalfi AN, et al. Acellular dermis-assisted prosthetic breast reconstruction versus complete submuscular coverage: a head-to-head comparison of outcomes. Plast Reconstr Surg 2009;124(6):1736–40.

26. Spear SL, Parikh PM, Reisin E, et al. Acellular dermis-assisted breast reconstruction. Aesthetic Plast Surg 2008;32:418–25.

27. Topol BM, Dalton EF, Ponn T, et al. Immediate single-stage breast reconstruction using implants and human acellular dermal tissue matrix with adjustment of the lower pole of the breast to reduce unwanted lift. Ann Plast Surg 2008;61:494–9.

28. Uflacker AB, Janis JE. The use of acellular dermal matrix in the correction of visible parasternal deformities after breast reconstruction. Plast Reconstr Surg 2010;126(1):34e–6e.

29. Zienowicz RJ, Karacaoglu E. Implant-based breast reconstruction with allograft. Plast Reconstr Surg 2007;120:373–81.

30. Baxter RA. Intracapsular allogenic dermal grafts for breast implant-related problems. Plast Reconstr Surg 2003;112(6):1692–6 [discussion: 1697–8].

31. Brown RH, Izaddoost S, Bullocks JM. Preventing the "bottoming out" and "star-gazing" phenomena in inferior pedicle breast reduction with an acellular dermal matrix internal brassiere. Aesthetic Plast Surg 2010;34(6):760–7.

32. Curtis MS, Mahmood F, Nguyen MD, et al. Use of AlloDerm for correction of symmastia. Plast Reconstr Surg 2010;126(4):192e–3e.

33. Colwell AS, Breuing KH. Improving shape and symmetry in mastopexy with autologous or cadaveric dermal slings. Ann Plast Surg 2008;61(2):138–42.

34. Duncan DI. Correction of implant rippling using allograft dermis. Aesthet Surg J 2001;21(1):81–4.

35. Hartzell TL, Taghinia AH, Chang J, et al. The use of human acellular dermal matrix for the correction of secondary deformities after breast augmentation: results and costs. Plast Reconstr Surg 2010;126(5): 1711–20.

36. Maxwell GP, Gabriel A. Use of the acellular dermal matrix in revisionary aesthetic breast surgery. Aesthet Surg J 2009;29(6):485–93.

37. Mofid MM, Singh NK. Pocket conversion made easy: a simple technique using alloderm to convert subglandular breast implants to the dual-plane position. Aesthet Surg J 2009;29(1):12–8.

38. Spear SL, Seruya M, Clemens MW, et al. Acellular dermal matrix for the treatment and prevention of implant-associated breast deformities. Plast Reconstr Surg 2011;127(3):1047–58.

39. Newman MI, Swartz KA, Samson MC, et al. The true incidence of near-term postoperative complications

in prosthetic breast reconstruction utilizing human acellular dermal matrices: a meta-analysis. Aesthetic Plast Surg 2011;35(1):100–6.

40. Jansen L, Macadam SA. The use of AlloDerm in postmastectomy alloplastic breast reconstruction: part I. A systematic review. Plast Reconstr Surg 2011;127(6):2232–44.

41. Jansen L, Macadam SA. The use of AlloDerm in postmastectomy alloplastic breast reconstruction: part II. A cost analysis. Plast Reconstr Surg 2011; 127(6):2245–54.

42. De Blacam C, Momoh AL, Colakoglu S, et al. Cost analysis of implant-based breast reconstruction with acellular dermal matrix. Ann Plast Surg 2011. [Epub ahead of print].

43. Chew RT, Sprague S, Thoma A. A systematic review of utility measurements in the surgical literature. J Am Coll Surg 2005;200:954–64.

44. Russell LB, Gold MR, Siegel JE, et al. The role of cost-effectiveness analysis in health and medicine: Panel on Cost-Effectiveness in Health and Medicine. JAMA 1996;276(14):1172–7.

45. Weinstein MC, Siegel JE, Gold MR, et al. Recommendations of the Panel on Cost-Effectiveness in Health and Medicine. JAMA 1996;276(15):1253–8.

46. Thoma A, Sprague S, Tandan V. Users' guide to the surgical literature: how to use an article on economic analysis. Can J Surg 2001;44:347–54.

47. Kotsis SV, Chung KC. Fundamental principles of conducting a surgery economic analysis study. Plast Reconstr Surg 2010;125(2):727–35.

48. Drummond MF, Richardson WS, O'Brien BJ, et al. Users' guide to the medical literature: XIII. How to use an article on economic analysis of clinical practice. A. Are the results of the study valid? Evidence-Based Medicine Working Group. JAMA 1997;277:1552.

49. Drummond MF, O'Brien BJ, Stoddart GL, et al. Methods for the economic evaluation of health care programmes. 2nd edition. Oxford (United Kingdom): Oxford University Press; 1997.

50. Siegel JE, Weinstein MC, Russell LB. Recommendations for reporting cost-effectiveness analyses. JAMA 1996;276(16):1339–41.

51. Wainright DJ. The use of an allograft dermal matrix (AlloDerm) in the management of full thickness burns. Burns 1995;21(4):243–8.

52. Tal H. Subgingival acellular dermal matrix allograft for the treatment of gingival recession: a case report. J Periodontol 1999;70(9):1118–24.

53. Shorr N, Perry JD, Goldberg RA, et al. The safety and applications of acellular human dermal allograft in ophthalmic plastic and reconstructive surgery: a preliminary report. Ophthal Plast Reconstr Surg 2000;16(3):223–300.

54. Sclafani AP, Romo T 3rd, Jacono AA, et al. Evaluation of acellular dermal graft in sheet (AlloDerm) and injectable (micronized AlloDerm) forms for soft tissue augmentation. Clinical observations and histological analysis. Arch Facial Plast Surg 2000; 2(2):120–36.

55. Buinewicz B, Rosen B. Acellular cadaveric dermis (AlloDerm): a new alternative for abdominal hernia repair. Ann Plast Surg 2004;52(2):188–94.

56. An G, Walter RJ, Nagy K. Closure of abdominal wall defects using acellular dermal matrix. J Trauma 2004;56(6):1266–75.

57. Terino EO. Alloderm acellular dermal graft: applications in aesthetic soft-tissue augmentation. Clin Plast Surg 2001;28:83–99.

58. Chaplin JM, Constantino PD, Wolpoe ME. Use of an acellular dermal allograft for dural replacement: an experimental study. Neurosurgery 1999; 16:196–201.

59. Livesey SA, Herndon DN, Hollyoak MA, et al. Transplanted acellular allograft dermal matrix: potential as a template for the reconstruction of viable dermis. Transplantation 1995;60:1.

60. Eppley BL. Experimental assessment of the revascularization of acellular human dermis for soft tissue augmentation. Plast Reconstr Surg 2001;107:757.

61. Menon NG, Rodriguez ED, Byrnes CK, et al. Revascularization of human acellular dermis in full-thickness abdominal wall reconstruction in the rabbit model. Ann Plast Surg 2003;50(5):523–7.

62. Campbell KT, Burns NK, Rios CN, et al. Human non-cross-linked porcine acellular dermal matrix used for ventral hernia repair: comparison of in vivo fibrovascular remodeling and mechanical repair strength. Plast Reconstr Surg 2011;127(6):2321–32.

63. Xu H, Wan H, Sandor M, et al. Host response to human acellular dermal matrix transplantation in a primate model of abdominal wall repair. Tissue Eng Part A 2008;14(12):2009–19.

64. Stump A, Holton LH, Connor J, et al. The use of acellular dermal matrix to prevent capsule formation around implants in a primate model. Plast Reconstr Surg 2009;124(1):82–91.

65. Uzunismail A, Duman A, Perk C, et al. The effects of acellular dermal allograft (AlloDerm) interface on silicone related capsule formation-experimental study. Eur J Surg 2008;31(4):170–85.

66. Basu CB, Leong M, Hicks J. Does Acellular Cadaveric Dermis (ACD) affect breast implant capsule formation in reconstructive breast surgery? A histopathologic comparison of breast capsule and ACD. Plast Reconstr Surg 2010;126(6):1842–7.

67. Wei ES, Lesperance M, Speers CH, et al. Increased use of regional radiotherapy is associated with improved outcome in a population based cohort of women with breast cancer with 1-3 positive nodes. Radiother Oncol 2010;97(2):301–6.

68. Kronowitz SJ, Robb GL. Breast reconstruction with postmastectomy radiation therapy: current issues. Plast Reconstr Surg 2004;114(4):950–60.

69. Lee BT, Adesiyun T, Colakoglu S, et al. Postmastec-tomy radiation therapy and breast reconstruction: and analysis of complication and patient satisfaction. Ann Plast Surg 2009;62(4):350–4.

70. Spear SL, Oneyewu C. Staged breast reconstruction with saline filled implants in the irradiated breast: recent trends and therapeutic implications. Plast Reconstr Surg 2000;105(3):930–42.

71. Dubin MG, Feldman M, Ibrahim HZ, et al. Allograft dermal implant (AlloDerm) in a previously irradiated field. Laryngoscope 2000;110(6):934–7.

72. Ibrhaim HZ, Kwiatkowski TJ, Montone KT, et al. Effects of external beam radiation on the allograft dermal implant. Otolaryngol Head Neck Surg 2000;122(2):189–94.

73. Komorowska-Timek E, Oberg KC, Timek TA, et al. The effect of AlloDerm envelopes on periprosthetic capsule formation with and without radiation. Plast Reconstr Surg 2009;123(3):807–16.

74. Available at: http://www.allergan.com/assets/pdf/L034-03_silicone_DFU.pdf. Accessed August 1, 2011.

75. Available at: http://www.mentorwwwlc.com/pdf/approved/gel-PIDS.pdf. Accessed August 1, 2011.

76. Maxwell GP, Gabriel A. The neopectoral pocket in revisionary breast surgery. Aesthet Surg J 2008;28:463–7.

77. Maxwell GP, Gabriel A. Efficacy of the neopectoral pocket in revisionary breast surgery. Aesthet Surg J 2009;29:379–85.

78. Chasan PE. Breast capsulorrhaphy revisited: a simple technique for complex problems. Plast Reconstr Surg 2005;115:296–301.

79. Hammond DC, Hidalgo D, Slavin SA, et al. Revising the unsatisfactory breast augmentation. Plast Reconstr Surg 1999;104:277–83.

80. Spear SL, Dayan JH, West J. The anatomy of revisions after primary breast augmentation: one surgeon's perspective. Clin Plast Surg 2009;36:157–65.

81. Spear SL, Bogue DP, Thomassen JM. Synmastia after breast augmentation. Plast Reconstr Surg 2006;118(Suppl 7):168S–71S.

Index

Note: Page numbers of article titles are in **boldface** type.

plasticsurgery.theclinics.com